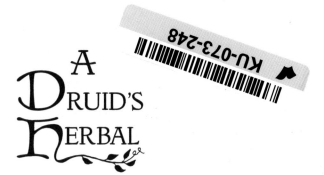

A Druid's Herbal

FOR THE
SACRED
EARTH YEAR

ALSO BY ELLEN EVERT HOPMAN

Tree Medicine, Tree Magic

Gifts of the Healing Earth Vol I (video)

Pagans (video)

A DRUID'S HERBAL

FOR THE SACRED EARTH YEAR

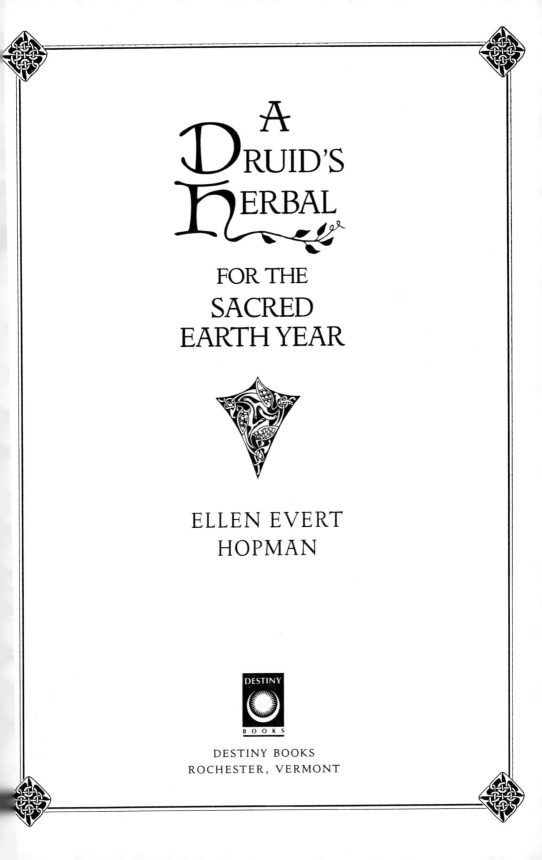

ELLEN EVERT
HOPMAN

DESTINY
BOOKS

DESTINY BOOKS
ROCHESTER, VERMONT

Destiny Books
One Park Street
Rochester, Vermont 05767
www.InnerTraditions.com

LIBRARY OF CONGRESS CATALOGING-IN-PUBLICATION DATA

Hopman, Ellen Evert.
    A druid's herbal for the sacred earth year / by Ellen Evert Hopman.
        p.   cm.
    Includes bibliographical references and index.
    ISBN 0-89281-501-9
    1. Druids and Druidism—Miscellanea. 2. Herbs—Religious aspects.
3. Religious calendars—Paganism. 4. Paganism—Rituals. I. Title.
BL910.H56   1994
299.16–dc20   94–4412
                                                                  CIP

Printed and bound in the United States

10 9 8 7 6 5

Text design by Virginia L. Scott
Layout by Electric Dragon Productions
Illustrations on pages 4 and 20 by Dan Mendoza
This book was typeset in Palantino with Charlemagne and Barbara Svelte as
    display typefaces

Destiny Books is a division of Inner Traditions International

---

Please note: In the event of a medical situation, readers are advised to seek the assistance of a competent health professional. Many of the remedies described in this book are based on herbal tradition and have not necessarily been empirically proven. Persons on medications prescribed by a health professional should seek advice before ingesting herbal preparations. The author may be contacted at P.O. Box 219, Amherst, MA 01004.

A dhaoine Sidhe;
A Tuatha Dé Danann;
Beannachtaí Dé Danann oraibh aqus orainn

O People of the Sidhe;
O Peoples of the Goddess Dana;
The blessings of the Goddess Dana upon you and upon us.

ACKNOWLEDGMENTS

Some of the formulas are based on research rather than personal experience. Readers' comments are welcome and encouraged.

My grateful thanks to Anna Kirwan-Vogel for her patient and thoughtful editing and to Emma Leah Tailleir, Paul Eagle, and Margaret Howe for their computer wizardry. Thanks are due to Dr. Paul Eric Smith for assistance with the Latin taxonomy. Many thanks to Stewart Farrar for permission to use the blessing that appears in the dedication.

Buíochas le hEadhmonn Ua Cuinn as ucht sleachta as Gaelige atá in úsáid sa leabhar seo. Go raibh maith agat Alexei Kondratiev for deepening my appreciation of the Celtic mysteries.

To Brighid, Patroness of the Druids and Bards

Beloved Brighid of the triple flame,
Daughter of the Dagda,
Guardian of the sacred springs
Whose voice is the soul of the harp
We call on Thee.
Teach our hands to heal and our hearts to sing.
We entrust our life's progress to your care
and ask that you shape us,
bending and turning our hearts on your bright anvil of flame
till we are made perfect jewels
fit to be set in the Eye of your timeless harp
to play for the Soul of the people in times of sorrow
and times of celebration.
We thank you for your gifts to us of Poetry and Music
of laughter and tears,
and for the healing balm of your Wisdom.
May we always remember to meditate
on the gift of your sacred waters,
which surround us at our birth
and sail us to our destiny.
Our hearts are open to receive your blessings.
Midwife of our souls, rain on us,
shower your inspiration in curtains of song
from sacred waterfalls in the realm where you dwell.
Come to us as Virgin with the soft smell of flowers.
Come to us as Mother and feed us your fruits.
Come to us as the Wise Woman in the stark blasts of Winter.
Help us to see your Mystery in all creation,
that we may know gratitude and reverence.
Our hearts sing to you with love.
Teach us to change like the revolving seasons.
Teach us to grow like the green corn that feeds the people.
Teach us to fashion beauty like the stillness of the forest pool
and the roar of the ocean wave.
Teach us to heal like the soothing gem which cools the eyes and
restores the limbs.
With humility and bright expectation
We invoke Thee this hour!

Contents

Introduction

"Thou shalt not suffer a witch to live" (Exod. 22:18) is the Biblical injunction most often used to condemn those who practice the ancient Earth religions. Biblical scholars, however, will attest that before the King James Version of the Bible, scripture would have read "thou shalt not suffer a *poisoner* to live."

Imagine the course of history if that injunction had been heeded. Instead of burning helpless women and men, the inquisitors might have gone after the industries and individuals who poison the water, the air, and the Earth and her children.

Modern folk have at last begun to contemplate the effects of ignoring nature in science, in daily life, and in religion. Too long have we been viewing the Earth as "God's footstool." Human civilization begins to look like a creeping cancer: cells out of control, each person going his or her own way ignoring the needs of other living beings. It is time to stop and begin again to honor the Earth and her rhythms.

How to begin? Sometimes the most moving ritual is one performed alone, sitting on the Earth, singing to a tree or a stone, dancing beneath the moon and sky, offering a gift of herbs to the sacred directions.

This is a book designed to inspire solitary and communal activities. My belief is that the Old Way must and will be the way of the future, if we are to have one. May these pages go forth as a blessing to the sun kings and queens, the fully illumined ones. May our efforts reopen the walls between the worlds until these, our elder brothers and sisters, walk with us again. May their light pierce the dark of the shadows that have too long held us apart. By the Three Worlds may this be so.

The central myth of the herbal healer is the story of Diancecht and his son Miach. Diancecht, the God of medicine, became jealous when his son's reputation as a healer eclipsed his own. Diancecht called for his son and hit him on the head with a sword. Miach easily healed himself. Diancecht struck him again, cutting him to the very bone. Miach cured himself a second time. Then the father struck his son's skull through to the brain, but Miach was able to heal himself once more. Finally, Diancecht cleaved Miach's brain in two, and this time the son died.

Diancecht buried his son, and thrice hundred and sixty-five herbs emerged from Miach's body. Each one was a cure for the illnesses of the three hundred sixty-five nerves of the human body. (This is probably a reference to a now lost astronomical plant classification system.)

Airmid, Miach's sister, carefully gathered the herbs and arranged them on her cloak in the shape of a human to denote their properties and show where they were useful in the human body. Diancecht, ever jealous, kicked the cloak and scattered the herbs, confusing their positions. If it hadn't been for his actions, we moderns would know the cure for every illness and we would be immortal, according to the ancients.

Hidden in this mystery lies the mystical secret of the herbal healer's art. The green herbs of the fields represent the body of the God (the Green Man), which is sacred and immortal. When an herbalist gathers herbs, she or he is dismembering the God, and when administering them to the body that is sick, she is ritually reuniting the lost pieces of the God and bringing the world back into wholeness.

Written on the full moon in Cutios (March) 1991 C.E.

CHAPTER 1

The Druids

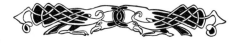

Who were the Druids? The ancient poet-priests and -priestesses who have inspired so much reverence and so much nonsense since they were replaced by Christianity in the fifth century C.E. have been credited with the building of Stonehenge (not true), with being Atlanteans (no evidence), and with being a lost tribe of Israel (doubtful). Eighteenth-century romantics such as John Toland and Henry Hurle (both Freemasons) have bequeathed to us the image of the white-garbed, bearded, male priest with a sickle.

History has generally chosen to ignore the ancients' testimony to the existence of female Druids—whole islands of them—and Tacitus' description of the black-clad screaming Druidesses who attempted to fight off the Romans at Anglesey in 61 C.E.

The Irish archdruid was described by his contemporaries as wearing the skin of a white bull and a white-feathered headdress with fluttering wings, or a many-colored cloak and ornaments of gold.* The white robes we moderns envision were worn for specific rituals such as gathering sacred herbs.

The Tain Bo Cuailnge is an ancient Gaelic tale from the La Tene (Iron Age) pre-Roman civilization. It is the oldest vernacular epic in Western literature. From it, we can glean some references to the Druids and their

---

*For an excellent overview of the archaeological and written evidence see Anne Ross, *Pagan Celtic Britain*.

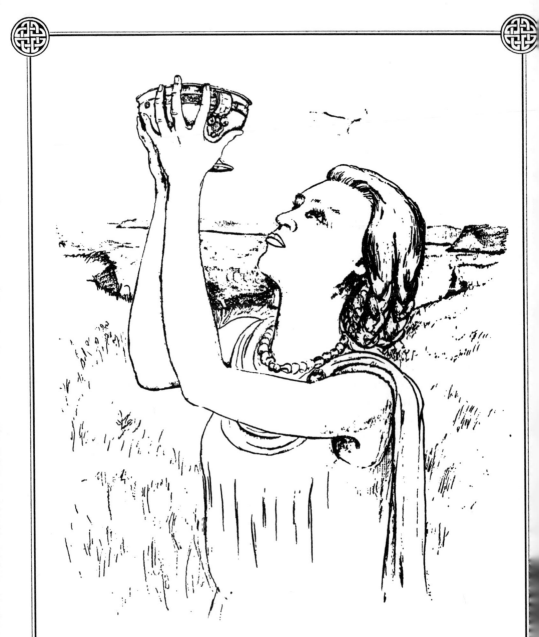

In this drawing a Druidess or Druid Priestess makes an offering to the Sun Goddess. The chalice she holds is of the ancient style, as are her knotted hair, her brooch, and her torque—symbolic of her rank. She does this in the presence of Land, Sea, and Sky—the three worlds of the ancient Celts, which were associated with (respectively) Nature Spirits, the Ancestors, and the Deities.

functions. According to the Tain, Druids could shape-change into deer and prophesy the future.

The Tain also gives us some idea of the ancient healing practices used by the Iron Age Celts. The hero CuChulainn healed the wounded Morrigan by wishing her health and by placing the blessings of the gods and the non-gods upon her. Lug mac Ethnenn, one of the sidhe (fairies), sang CuChulainn to sleep for three days and nights that his wounds might heal. He then dropped healing herbs and grasses into the sores while CuChulainn slept.

Other healers are described as dropping plants and herbs into the wounds of Ferdia as well. Charioteers made beds of fresh rushes with headrests for the wounded.

Serious wounds that spurted blood had magic amulets laid on them, and spells and incantations were sung over them by healers. The wounded CuChulainn was bathed in numerous streams and rivers to restore his health after battle. His wounds were bound with hazel twigs. The mortally wounded Cethern was made to sleep day and night in bone marrow.

Other legends tell us that the Druids could raise winds and fogs, dry up lakes and rivers, and lay hills flat.

The Druids did not use formal buildings for their religious services. Their sanctuaries were the Nemetons: cleared spaces in a forest, surrounded by earthworks, a wooden palisade, or trees. The teachings of the Druids, which could take up to twenty years to impart, were given in forests away from the distractions of hill forts or towns.

The word "Druid" most likely comes from the prefix *dru*, meaning "hard, true, resistant, permanent." *Dru-uides* were the "true-seers," and the word for a female Druid was *ban-drui*, or Druidess. Druids studied divination, magic, astrology, theology, law, medicine, natural sciences, music, and poetry. So well respected were they that they advised queens and kings.

The teachings of the Druids were passed down orally; very little was written. This was not, however, for want of an alphabet. The ancient Celts used *ogham*, or the "tree alphabet," for secular matters, preferring to keep the important Druidic knowledge sacred and less accessible by committing it to memory. Gaulish Druids went to Britain for formal training but met in France at Chartres, at the site of the present-day cathedral.

Within the Druid orders, Brehons, Vates, and Bards had separate functions. Bards specialized in poetic composition and singing, whereas the Vates practiced divination and seership. The Brehons were the judges, arbiters of the ancient Brehon laws. The clergy—priests and priestesses—were referred to as "Druids."

Both Bards and Druids could arbitrate in wars and could even stop a battle. The Brehons presided over criminal, civil, and property disputes. They were empowered to put individuals to death for serious offenses, much as we do today. A severe judgement could bar an individual from religious rites, thus stripping them of both secular and religious status. Druids could invoke divine retribution upon an individual or a tribe by ritual cursing.

According to Pliny the Druids reckoned the beginning of each month on the sixth day following the new moon. The day began at twilight, as darkness was understood to precede light, much as gestation precedes birth and chaos precedes creation.

Druids were the history-keepers, the repositories of lore and wisdom. They were "living books." Law, medicine, the knowledge of nature and the gods and goddesses, the Otherworld, and the timing of ritual and agricultural cycles were their special domain.

THE BARDS

The Bards were the storytellers. It was their duty to hold forth at ceremonial occasions, such as night vigils at holy wells; after religious services; at wakes, baby blessings, weddings, and house blessings; before battles; at the serving of ale; and at feasts and inheritances. Before the start of a voyage, before a court appearance, and before a hunt were also auspicious times for a tale.

The subjects of the stories were typically suited to the occasion. "Battle" stories were told before going to war, "cattle-raids" before raiding cattle, "voyages" before starting out to sea, "conceptions and births" at baby blessings, "wooings" at weddings, "death tales" at wakes, and so on.

In the Book of Leinster and other sources, lists appear of types of stories such as "Destructions" (*Tógála*), "Battles" (*Catha*), "Feasts" (*Fessa*), "Elopements" (*Aithid*), "Visions" (*Fisi*), "Loves" (*Serca*), "Voyages" (*Immrama*), "Sieges" (*Forbassa*), "Conceptions and Births" (*Coimperta*)

and "Frenzies" (*Buili*), etc. At the great assemblies many types of tales were told together.

The Bards were the keepers of the heroic cycles and of rhymes, riddles, songs, prayers, proverbs, traditions, and genealogical lore. Sacred stories could be recited only at night between Samhain (Halloween) and Beltaine (May Day). The center of Bardic activity was often the hearth, the "fire altar" at the heart of the home.

In Ireland, a master poet (*Ollamh*) was equal to a king under the law. She or he practiced divination and prophecy and, wearing a cloak of bird feathers, used ritual and trance to take listeners to the Otherworld. Hearing the stories was more than entertainment. Those who listened attentively were promised health, wealth, progeny, freedom from captivity, safe voyage, and protection.

Let it never be forgotten that the storyteller's art was a sacred Druidic function. The ancient Welsh word for story, *cyfarwyddyd*, meant also "guidance," "direction," "instruction," "prescription," "knowledge," and "skill." The word *arwydd*, from which it is derived, means "sign," "symbol," "omen," and "miracle"; at its root is the word "to see." The *cyfarwydd* were thus guides to the Otherworld; to the sacred, mysterious meanings behind things; and to the great lessons of history.

In Wales, the chief poet (*pencerdd*) was as highly positioned socially as the highest officials at court. Under him in rank was the household poet (*bardd teulu*), who was given his harp from the king's hand and kept it for life. The duties of a household poet were to inspire the troops before a battle and to compose love poems. The *cerddorion* (minstrels) were a third class of poets under the pencerdd.

The duties of minstrels and poets generally were to encourage the people, to make them happy, and to inspire generosity. When the master poets began to die out the function of the Bards degenerated to the composing of praise-poems.

At royal functions, the king or queen, the heir to the throne, the chief judge, and the chief poet sat together, while the royal guard and the household bard sat below. If the king or queen desired music, the chief bard would sing twice in the upper hall and a song from the household bard in the lower hall would follow. The household bard also sang for the queen in her chambers.

The poets had a fearful weapon at their disposal: satire. It was a terrible thing to be subjected to Bardic wrath, which could make animals and land barren and cause the face to erupt into blisters.

An Ollamh, or master poet, was one who could recite three hundred and fifty stories. To perfect their art and to increase their sensory acuity, the poets would study in darkness or lie on the ground with stones on their stomachs and cloths wrapped about their heads until they had composed a poem.

One of the three Brighids is patroness of the Bards. The other two manifestations of this triple goddess are a healer and a smith.

THE OVATES

Ovates, or Vates, were the keepers of prophecy, divination, and sacrifice. They were the ones who dispatched the prisoners of war and the criminal outcasts. Four forms of death were meted out by these sacrificers: death by air (hanging), death by water (drowning), death by fire (cremation), and death by earth (burial alive). The triple death of air, water, and earth was used for ritual sacrifice and to punish oathbreakers.

While it is true that ancient Druids practiced sacrifices, we have no evidence that the descriptions offered by Julius Caesar of burning wicker holocausts are to be trusted. Caesar was, after all, attempting to get money from Rome so that he could further his political ambitions. He was probably engaging in propaganda as he described the "vicious" sacrifices of the Druids to the Romans of the bread and circus.

Modern-day Druids most emphatically *do not* engage in the harm or sacrifice of any living thing.

BELIEFS

The most basic doctrine of the Druids was and is the belief in reincarnation. Beyond that there are some religious and philosophical tenets that set Druids apart from other neo-Pagan systems of thought and practice, such as Wicca or witchcraft.

The Druids were and are polytheistic. Gods and goddesses each hold special functions all their own, and individual goddesses are often described as triple or trinitarian in nature.

The number three is of paramount importance: the Three Worlds of water (ancestors, the Otherworld), land (earthly beings), and sky (deities) are significant, as are the three foundations of the Bardic art: sound, speech, and music. The past and future are constantly related through the present. Two opposites are harmonized by the introduction of a third force or element. The sun, moon, and earth are a basic trilogy, as is the concept of sound, light and power that manifest as form.

Some have speculated that the Druid religion had its origins in ancient India, where the emphasis was on fire worship and on a threefold divinity: Brahma (creator), Shiva (destroyer), and Vishnu (sustainer).

For whatever reason, the sacred triad remains a basic building block, the trilithon of the Druidic mystery.

The Coligny Calendar of the Gaulish Druids

One of the very few remaining examples of Druid writing and culture, the Coligny calendar, is a bronze tablet of the Gaulish Druids of the first century found at Bourg near Lyons, France. Discovered in 1897 in the tribal lands of the Sequani, it represents about three-fifths of the entire original work. A bronze statue was found with it, making it likely that its location was a public temple.

Sixty-two consecutive months are inscribed. Each month is depicted in a vertical arrangement of Roman numerals and letters. Most months are given five times, thus marking a cycle of five years.

The calendar is lunar, with six months of thirty days each and five months of twenty-nine days each. Individual months are labelled *matvs* (good) or *anmatvs* (not good), meaning "lucky" or "not lucky." Individual days are either D (*dij*) for "day" or MD (*matvs dij*) for "good day."

The days are reckoned from sunset to sunset, and the Druidical month seems to have begun on the sixth day from the appearance of the moon. This is the day upon which, Pliny tells us, the Druids used to gather mistletoe.

Each month was divided into a light half of fifteen days and a dark half of fourteen or fifteen days. The full moon fell on the seventh, eighth, or ninth day of the light half of the Druidical month. The new moon occurred at about the middle of the second (dark) half of each month.

At intervals of two and a half or three years an intercalary month of thirty days was added so this lunar calendar could be made to conform to the solar year. The month of Anagantios (February) was twenty-eight days long one year and thirty the next, in alternating sequence.

Though the calendar uses Roman script it is not related to the Roman way of timekeeping. The Roman calendar was not designed to follow natural events such as full moons or new moons.

The Druidical year was divided into two halves. From Samonios (October/November) to Giamonios (April/May) was the dark half of the year; from Giamonios to Samonios was the light half.

Certain festivals or holy days are marked on the calendar. The winter and summer solstices have special designations, as does an equivalent festival to Lugnasad and a festival at the same time as Beltaine. Interestingly, there is no special designation for Samhain or for Oimealg. Every few years in Rivros there seems to have been a great festival.

The calendar provides us with about sixty Celtic words, most of which are used to describe the character of individual days. For example, some days are "lifeless" or "barren"; other days are "good."

The names of the months are descriptions of the activities of the Celtic year. Simivisonios marks the "bright spring"; Edrinios, the "hot time." Elembivios is named after a wooden fence, marking the appropriate time to repair fences damaged by cattle. Equos was the time of horse racing or trading. Giamonios was the "shoots' time" or "winter's end." Samonios was the "seed time" or "summer's end."

Ogronios marked the "cool month," Cutios, the "time of winds." Dumannios was "dark." Rivros was "frost time," and Anagantios was "time to stay indoors." Cantlos was the "song month," perhaps to celebrate the harvest.*

The Months of the Coligny Calendar

Dark Half
Samonios   October/November
Dumannios   November/December
Rivros   December/January
Anagantios   January/February
Ogronios   February/March
Cutios   March/April

Light Half
Giamonios   April/May
Simivisonios   May/June
Equos   June/July
Elembivios   July/August
Edrinios   August/September
Cantlos   September/October

---

* For further details about the Coligny Calendar, please see Eoin MacNeill, "On the Calendar of Coligny."

THE CELTIC TREE CALENDAR
AND ALPHABET

The Irish ogham script, or tree alphabet, was in use, and the Celtic Tree Calendar may have been in use until 700 C.E. This calendar is a lunar calendar in which the months are reckoned from new moon to new moon.*

THE CELTIC TREE CALENDAR

Beith	Birch	November
Luis	Rowan	December
Fearn	Alder	January
Saille	Willow	February
Nuin	Ash	March
Huathe	Hawthorn	April
Duir	Oak	May
Tinne	Holly	June
Coll	Hazel	July
Quert	Apple	—
Muin	Vine	August
Gort	Ivy	September
Ngetal	Reed	October
Straif	Blackthorn	—
Ruis	Elder	Last three days of October

THE TREE ALPHABET

THE OGHAM

B	Beith	Birch	
L	Luis	Rowan	
F	Fearn	Alder	

---

* For a detailed description please see Liz and Colin Murray, *The Celtic Tree Oracle*, or Robert Graves, *The White Goddess*. (Many people believe that the Tree Calendar is a pure invention of the poet Robert Graves, who claims to have intuited the evidence.)

S	Saille	Willow	
N	Nuin	Ash	
H	Huathe	Hawthorn	
D	Duir	Oak	
T	Tinne	Holly	
C	Coll	Hazel	
Q	Quert	Apple	
M	Muin	Vine	
G	Gort	Ivy	
P or Ng	Pethboc/Ngetal	Dwarf Elder/Reed	
Ss	Straif	Blackthorn	
R	Ruis	Elder	
A	Ailim	Silver Fir	
O	Ohn	Furze	
U	Ur	Heather	
E	Eadha	White Poplar	
I	Ioho	Yew	
Y	Too sacred to have a written name	Mistletoe	

The ogham alphabet was used to carve names onto the edges of standing stones and to send messages on sticks of wood.

CHAPTER 2

Herbal Basics

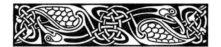

The physician does not learn everything he must know and master at high college alone; from time to time he must consult old women, gypsies, magicians, wayfarers, and all manner of peasant folk and random people, and learn from them; for these have more knowledge about such things than all the high colleges. . . . Therefore study each day without respite, investigate and observe diligently; despise nothing, and do not lightly put too much trust in yourself. Do not be arrogant when in fact you are helpless, and do not regard yourself as a master at the outset; for no one can achieve mastery without labor. Also, learn from those who are more experienced than you, for who can pretend to know everything? Who can be everywhere and know where all things lie? Therefore travel and explore everything, and whatever comes your way, take it without scorn and do not be ashamed to do so. . . . For nature is so excellent in its gifts that . . . it better benefit a man to know one herb in the meadow, but to know it thoroughly, than to see the whole meadow without knowing what grows on it.

Paracelsus

HERBAL PREPARATIONS

Whether you intend to tincture or dry your herbs, a few basic rules apply.

Tree leaves should be gathered before Midsummer. After that, the percentage of natural insecticide in the leaf is too high.

Leaves and flowers are gathered on a dry day when the flowers first begin to open. They are always dried in the shade.

Roots are generally gathered in very early spring or in late fall after the plant has begun to die back.

Tree barks generally contain the desired medicinal properties in the soft inner layer (cambium) between the sapwood and the dead outer bark, or the bark of the root.

GENERAL RULES FOR HERBAL PREPARATIONS

When Using Leaves or Flowers

Steep two teaspoons per cup of water for about twenty minutes. Strain and store in a refrigerated, airtight container. The dose is one-fourth of a cup four times a day, not with meals. Children take one-eighth cup, and infants can receive the herbs through the mother's milk.

When Using Roots, Barks, Seeds and Twigs

Simmer two teaspoons of plant matter for twenty minutes, strain, and store as above. The dose is one-fourth cup, four times a day, not with meals.

Herbal teas will stay fresh in your refrigerator for about one week when stored in an airtight container.

HERBAL DOSAGES

The dosages indicated in the "Herbal Uses" section under each herb assume that the patient is a 150-pound adult. Children (75 pounds) receive one-half the indicated amount. Infants (25 pounds) receive a one-quarter dose, and newborns can get a dose through the mother's breast milk. The usual dose for a formula or tea is one-quarter cup three or four times a day, and not with meals.

SALVES

Herbs that are useful for skin conditions (such as comfrey, lavender, calendula, pine needles, aloes, elecampane root, burdock, and elderflowers) can be made into salves. The ideal time to make a salve is summer, when the herbs are fresh and abundant, but dried herbs can be used as well. I like to add green walnut hulls and whole, smashed horse chestnuts to the basic mix for their skin-healing and painkilling virtues.

Simmer herbs in good quality olive oil in a large pot. In a separate pot, melt and simmer three to four tablespoons of fresh beeswax (the beeswax should be of a golden color with a strong honey scent) per cup of oil. Put enough oil in the pot to just cover the herbs. Simmer the herbs in the oil for about twenty minutes. When wax and oil reach the same temperature, pour in the wax. Strain and pour into clean jars. Tincture of benzoin (about one ounce per quart) may be added as a preservative while the salve is still liquid although it is not strictly necessary. The most important factor in controlling mold is to have immaculately clean and dry jars and utensils. Boiling followed by thorough drying is all that is usually needed. Persons living in very hot and damp climates may want to take the extra precaution of adding the tincture of benzoin.

TINCTURES

Tinctures are made by grinding the leaves, roots, or other plant parts with a mortar and pestle (or a blender) and just barely covering them with high-quality vodka, whiskey, or grain alcohol. After twenty-one days, add a small quantity of glycerine (about two tablespoons per pint) and about 10 percent per volume of spring water. Strain and store in amber glass airtight containers. Keep the herbal tinctures in a cool, dry place for up to five years.

The dose is generally twenty drops in a cup of herb tea or warm water four times a day. In acute or emergency situations the dose is given more frequently; in the case of labor pains, for example, it might be a dropperful every five minutes.

POULTICES

To make a poultice take fresh herbs or dried ones that have been soaked in freshly boiled water until soft. Mix them with just enough slippery elm powder to make the poultice stick together. Place it on the affected part and wrap with a clean cloth. For added protection from staining, clear plastic wrap can be wrapped around the poultice and cloth.

FOMENTATIONS

A fomentation is a strong herbal tea in which a clean cloth is dipped (the cloth can also be filled with herbs). The cloth is then applied to the affected part.

SYRUPS

Syrups are made by boiling three pounds of Sucanat (dessicated sugar cane juice) in one pint of water until a syrupy consistency is obtained and then steeping the herbs in the hot mixture for twenty minutes. The herbs can also be simmered directly in honey or maple syrup for about ten minutes. Use two teaspoons of herb for every cup of liquid. Strain the syrup and store it, well sealed, in the refrigerator.

HOMEOPATHIC REMEDIES

Note: Homeopaths use herbs in *potentized* form. Homeopathic remedies are extremely dilute versions of herbal tinctures prepared by trituration and sucussion. The remedies are so dilute that any preparation with the potency of 30C or higher will have no molecule of the original substance left, and yet the medicines still bear a unique molecular "signature" as evidenced by nuclear resonance testing. For this reason herbs and other substances which might be poisonous in material doses are given with no ill effects. The homeopath selects a remedy based on the "symptom picture." Mental, emotional, and physical characteristics are examined and a remedy is selected that matches the person's unique configuration.

HOMEOPATHIC DOSAGES

Over-the-counter homeopathic remedies tend to be sold in the lower potencies (6X, 6C, 12X, or 12C). Professional homeopaths will tend to use the higher potencies (30C, 200C, 1M, 10M, etc.). The lower potencies are safer for home care of acute (short-term) conditions. In general, homeopathic remedies are repeated more often (every hour or two hours) when given for acute conditions. Constitutional prescribing— prescribing that takes the whole person (dietary preferences, exercise habits, emotional outlook, sleep, dreams, reproductive strength, allergies and sensitivities, history of illness, etc.) into account—may indicate a single dose of a higher potency. See the bibliography for some books on homeopathic medicine.

SUGGESTED MAGICAL USES OF HERBS

Herb magic can be thought of as a way of fixing one's conscious and unconscious mind on a universal energy pattern as it manifests in the plant kingdom. For example, white jasmine is a feminine, lunar herb of the element water. When ingested, she creates erotic emotions. For this reason, jasmine is an herb of choice for a love spell.

Spells are best worked at the waxing or full moon (unless you are attempting to banish something, in which case the waning moon is more appropriate). To work a simple spell, you need only call in the sacred directions* and then bury your herbs in the earth, cast them to living waters (a lake, pond, stream, or river, or the ocean), cast them to the air, cast them to the moon, or burn them so that the smoke can carry your intent to the winds. Then, simply thank the directions and know that your spell has been activated.

Sometimes, it is appropriate to carry an herb with you. For example, you might keep an acorn in your pocket to bring fertility to your creative acts. You might keep a certain herb (cinquefoil) in your house or bedroom to bless and protect the home. At other times, you may ritually sweep an area with an herb (juniper) to clear out negative energies, or you may wish to burn an herb (sage, frankincense) for its purifying scent as you set up your altar.

The essence of an herbal ritual is in the reverence and intent that you bring to it. Choose your herbs with care, and always leave a gift for the earth when you take one of her plant children: a pinch of vervain, tobacco, or corn meal, or a gift of new honey or cider.

Always remember the debt we owe to our green sisters and brothers. Without them, there would be no air to breathe and no food to sustain the Earth's creatures, including ourselves.

The Earth Festivals of the Sacred Earth Year

Samhain (All Hallows)	1 November
Meán Geimhridh (Winter Solstice, Yule)	21 December
Imbolg/Oimealg (Candlemas)	1 February
Meán Earraigh (Spring Equinox)	21 March
Beltaine (May Eve)	1 May
Meán Samhraidh (Summer Solstice, Midsummer)	21 June
Lugnasad (Lammas)	1 August
Meán Fómhair (Fall Equinox)	21 September

---

* Druids will want to call in the four directions and a fifth—the center. Please see Chapter 13, "Sacred Groves and Circles," for a further discussion of this practice.

Some folk prefer to celebrate the fire festivals (Samhain, Imbolc, Beltaine, Lugnasad) at the nearest full moon. Groups often find it convenient to celebrate on the nearest weekend. Private observances, however, should be performed on the actual day.

The herbs and other plants mentioned in the following festival observances are those in current neo-Pagan usage. Corn, potatoes, and pumpkins, for example, although unknown to the ancient Celts, have found contemporary uses. For a discussion of historically accurate herbal uses, please refer to chapter 11, "Herbs of the Druids."

CHAPTER 3

Samhain
All Hallows, the Celtic New Year

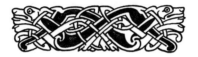

I had my days with kings,
Drinking mead and wine:
To-day I drink whey-water
Among the shriveled old hags.

from Dillon, **Early Irish Literature**

Deep-red the bracken, its shape all gone—
The wild goose has raised his wonted cry.
Cold has caught the wings of birds;
Season of ice—these are my tidings

from Dillon, **Early Irish Literature**

The Samhain festival falls at the end of the harvest and marks the conclusion of the agricultural cycle. At Samhain, the dark winter half of the year commences. It is the Celtic new year, the time when the walls between the worlds are thin, and communication is easy with those who have "passed over"—the wandering dead. It is a magical interval when the laws of time and space are suspended. Humans engage in strange and unpredictable behaviors that mirror the activities of the spirit world.

Samhain is the time to bring honor and hospitality to dead ancestors. Prayers and food offerings are left on doorsteps and altars. Even if they are untouched by morning, the essence of the food is said to be transferred to the spirits.

19

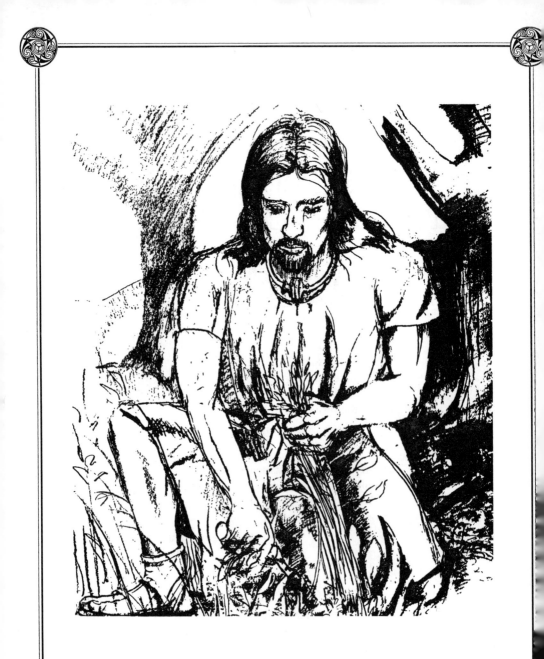

A young Druid priest ritually gathers the last sheaf of grain from the harvest. He is wearing a torque, symbol of his rank, and the white robes described by Roman witnesses. As he gathers the sheaf he meditates on the sacrifice of the grain god who has given his life so that all may eat.

Samhain is a time to slaughter cattle and in general to complete the unfinished business of summer. Any produce left in the fields after Samhain is taboo, as it now belongs to the nature spirits.

The new year begins at sunset on October 31. It marks a time of settling and reckoning of accounts, a time to finish with and discard influences and concepts that have outlived their usefulness. It is especially a time to reconnect with tribal and personal ancestors and guiding spirits.

Samhain is one of the two "spirit-nights" of the year (Beltaine being the other)—a time of chaos when the fairies are most active. It is a night when witches are about, omens are seen, divinations are made, and household fires are kindled anew.

At Samhain, the Sidhe-mounds open and the Sidhe are abroad in the countryside. The souls of the dead return and are made visible. It is a good time to clean the house and hearth in preparation for the visits of dead ancestors. Doors should be left unbolted and extra chairs put out.

To celebrate the darkness of the unborn year, traditional people dressed in white or donned straw disguises. Boys and girls exchanged clothing, and efforts were made to fool the wandering spirits. In the spirit of mischief and chaos that reigned generally, household items were sometimes stolen and tossed into ponds or ditches. Livestock could be led into other people's fields, and doors pelted with cabbages. Chimneys might be blocked with turf, and smoke blown in through keyholes.

Tales of the supernatural were told from sunset until dawn, when the first cockcrow sent the spirits and the "little people" back to their dwellings. Marked stones were cast into the fires, and their condition upon retrieval in the morning showed the person's fortune for the coming year.

Household fires were relit from sacred bonfires started by friction, and people jumped through the flames for luck. The ashes were scattered in the fields, and blazing torches were carried around the boundaries to bless and protect the land. Potatoes* and apples were roasted and eaten as joyful dances were made around the sacred flames.

In areas where seaweed was gathered, folk would come together at Samhain to offer a cup of ale or a bowl of porridge to the god of the sea, asking for a bountiful harvest of seaweed to eat and to fertilize the soil. The ritual was especially powerful if done in a storm, ensuring a bountiful harvest of sea vegetation of the shore.

---

* Potatoes were added to the traditional diet after the discovery of South America by Europeans.

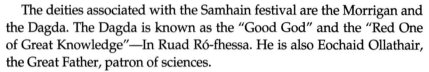

The deities associated with the Samhain festival are the Morrigan and the Dagda. The Dagda is known as the "Good God" and the "Red One of Great Knowledge"—In Ruad Ró-fhessa. He is also Eochaid Ollathair, the Great Father, patron of sciences.

Divine warrior and archetypal chieftain, the Dagda is the personification of fertility, generosity, lawgiving, and protection. He possesses a magical staff with which he can kill the living or resurrect the dead. He is owner of a huge cauldron from which healing, regeneration, and food are always available for the tribe.

The Dagda mated with the Morrigan as she straddled the River Unius in Connacht.

The Morrigan, or Great Queen, is a triple Goddess of the Celtic tradition. Her three facets are Badb (crow), Macha (also crow), and Nemain (frenzy). Known also as the Battle Crow, she appears in the shape of a crow or raven, or as a woman accompanied by one of these birds. Crows and ravens were once a common sight in battlefields as they arrived in flocks to pick the bones of dead warriors. The Morrigan is one who influences the course of battles and who prophesies their outcome. She sometimes appears at the riverside washing the weapons and equipment of those who are about to die.

At times she becomes a terrible hag dressed in red, or a surpassingly beautiful woman. If her amorous advances are rejected she becomes enraged, and she can shape-shift into an eel, a gray wolf, or a heifer—whichever form is most deadly to the offending suitor.

The Morrigan is markedly sexual. She is also a mother; she bore a son, Meiche, who had three hearts inhabited by three snakes capable of killing all the animals in Ireland. Diancecht, a god of healing, killed Meiche and burned the snakes, thus saving the land from disaster.

Badb, Macha, and Nemain, the three facets of the Morrigan, protected the Tuatha Dé Danaan with a cover of rain as they landed on Irish soil.

The Morrigan is maiden, mother, and crone. She is the cailleach (hag) who delights in bloody battles and in the drowning of enemy soldiers beneath the white-capped waves. She may at times appear in bright apparel edged with gold.

She is also the waxing, full, and waning moon, visible in the form of a raven to those about to die. Macha is the white foam on the ocean waves, the mane of the mother Morrigan's head. Daughter of the sea, she in honored with offerings at Samhain.

Samhain is, in essence, the time of preconception, the time of descent into black chaos from which new ideas and new life will ultimately spring.

THE HERBS OF SAMHAIN

Acorn and Oak, Apple, Arborvitae (Yellow Cedar), Corn, Dittany of Crete, Fumitory, Hazel, Mullein, Nightshade, Pumpkin, Sage, Turnip, Wormwood

Make an offering of cakes, cider, and song to some local fruit trees in thanks for the year's harvest.
Please refer to chapter 2, "Herbal Basics," for methods of preparation.

ACORN AND OAK, *QUERCUS* SPP.

Pliny says that acorns were roasted or dried and ground into flour to be made into bread. Acorns were also valued as pig fodder. Some species of acorns are bitter and must be leached in water before processing. (See also page 104 in "Herbs of the Druids.")

Parts Used: Inner bark (cambium) and young leaf; for the leaf, use two teaspoons per cup and steep for twenty minutes; for the bark, use one tablespoon per cup and simmer for twenty minutes.

Herbal Uses: The white oak (*Quercus alba*) is the best for internal use. Infuse the inner bark or young leaf (before Midsummer) for douches and enemas. Internal rectal problems, hemorrhoids, leukorrhea, menstrual irregularities, and bloody urine are also benefited. Take internally as a tea and apply externally in fomentation, to shrink varicose veins. The tea brings down fevers, treats diarrhea, and makes a wash for sores. Up to three cups a day may be safely taken. As a gargle, it treats mouth sores and sore throats. Being an astringent, it stops internal bleeding. Black oak (*Quercus tinctoria*) and red oak (*Quercus rubra*) can be used externally. English oak (*Quercus robur*) can be used both externally and internally.

Oak leaves are prepared in infusion for douches to treat vaginal infections; gather them *before* Midsummer. To prepare, steep one tablespoon per quart of water for thirty minutes. A tea of the buds is a valuable tonic for the liver; steep two teaspoons per cup of water for twenty minutes. Simmer the bark in salves to make a remedy for hemorrhoids; follow the general directions for salves on page 14.

Homeopathic Uses: Homeopaths use *Quercus glandium spiritus* (a tincture of acorns) for edema, splenetic dropsy, liver problems, and gout and to take away the craving for alcohol in alcoholics.

Magical Uses: The oak is a tree of the sun, and sacred to Brighid and the Dadga. Druids do not celebrate unless in the presence of an oak, yew, ash, or other sacred tree. Oak symbolizes abundance, fertility, longevity, protection, and the ability to withstand the lightning blasts of spiritual awareness while remaining firmly rooted in the material, or earth, plane. Oak is classic wood for staves and wands. All parts of the tree are powerful protective charms, which bring healing.

Acorns bring fertility and abundance to any endeavor. Carry one for good luck.

APPLE, *MALUS* SPP.

Parts Used: Whole apple (cooked or raw), apple cider, apple cider vinegar.

Herbal Uses: Apples clean the liver, cure constipation, and tone the gums. When baked they can be applied as a warm poultice to sore throats and skin inflammations. The cooked apple is especially laxative. The peeled raw apple helps with diarrhea. The cider corrects intestinal flora, reduces stomach acidity, corrects gas, and helps the kidneys; take three or four cups a day.

Apple cider vinegar and water make a rinse to restore hair, scalp, and skin; use equal parts of vinegar and water. Blondes should use white vinegar. Apple cider vinegar, water, and honey aid digestion when taken with meals; use two teaspoons of vinegar to a glass, add honey to taste.

Magical Uses: Apples as symbols of life and immortality are offered to the dead. They are buried at Samhain as food for those who are waiting to be reborn.

ARBORVITAE (YELLOW CEDAR), *THUJA OCCIDENTALIS*

Parts Used: Twig and leaf.

Herbal Uses: A member of the cypress family, cedar is used by herbalists to treat bloody cough and heart weakness. Simmer two teaspoons per cup for twenty minutes and take it cold in one-tablespoon doses, three to six times a day. It is used internally and externally as an antifungal (the dry powder is excellent for athlete's foot).

Homeopathic Uses: Homeopaths use *Thuja occidentalis* as an antibacterial agent and for the ill effects of vaccinations, gonorrhea, and warts. CAUTION: *Thuja should not be used by pregnant women.*

Magical Uses: The scent of cedar is said to allay grief. Known as a tree of immortality, it is used as a ritual herb in funerals. Cedar is burned with sage in traditional Native American "smudge sticks."

CORN, *ZEA MAYS*

Part Used: Fresh silk from organic plants.

Herbal Uses: Corn bread is more nutritious than wheat bread, and beans and corn together make a complete protein. Organic corn silk can be eaten fresh from the ears. It will tone the bladder; add it freely to salads. In winter it is available dried from herbalists, though the fresh silk has the best bladder-toning properties. Steep one teaspoon of the dried silk per cup of water for five minutes; take one tablespoon every two hours.

Homeopathic Uses: Homeopaths use *Stigmata Maydis-zea* (corn silk) for cystitis and kidney conditions, and *Ustilago maydis* (corn smut) for hemorrhage and lack of tone in the uterus.

Magical Uses: Corn on the altar represents the power of the Corn Mother, she who blesses and nourishes all of her earthly children.

DITTANY OF CRETE, *ORIGANUM DICTAMNUS*

Parts Used: Leaf, stem, and root.

Herbal Uses: Dittany leaf is simmered in ale or wine with vervain, hyssop, and pennyroyal to ease the pain of childbirth. Mix the herbs and simmer two teaspoons of the herbs per cup of liquid for twenty minutes; take up to two cups per day in half-cup doses. Simmer the herb or roots, using two tablespoons per cup, for twenty minutes. This can be applied to sprains, bruises, and rheumatism by means of a cloth fomentation.

Magical Uses: The scent of dittany is said to aid in astral projection.

FUMITORY, *FUMARIA OFFICINALIS*

Parts Used: Leaf and stem.

Herbal Uses: The warm infusion of the herb benefits eczema, dermatitis, and stomach and liver complaints. Taken over a long period, it helps to cure depression. Steep two teaspoons per cup for twenty minutes and drink the tea cold, a quarter cup four times a day. Tincture: twenty drops, four times a day.

Magical Uses: Fumitory is burned to exorcise unwanted spirit entities.

HAZEL, *CORYLUS AVELLANA*

Part Used: Nut.

Herbal Uses: Hazel nuts are rich in phosphorus, magnesium, potassium, and copper. Culpeper says that hazel nuts with mead or honey will cure a chronic cough. These are made into an "electuary." Grind the nuts in an electric blender, then add mead or honey to form a paste, which is eaten several times a day in tablespoon doses. Add pepper to discharge phlegm.

Magical Uses: Hazel is an ancient Celtic tree of wisdom, inspiration, and poetry. Hazel nuts are eaten before divination. The wood makes an excellent wand. The forked twigs are used by dowsers. Diancecht, the god of healing, invented a porridge that would cure colds, sore throats, and worms. According to legend, it consisted of hazel buds, dandelions, chickweed, sorrel, and oatmeal. It was to be taken in the mornings and evenings.

MULLEIN, *VERBASCUM THAPSUS*

Parts Used: Leaf and flower.

Herbal Uses: The leaf is a classic remedy for bronchitis (as well as other coughs) and burning urination. Simmer two teaspoons per cup and take a quarter cup four times a day. A tea of the flowers taken before bed brings on sleep. A poultice of the leaves helps wounds and sores; follow the general directions for poultices on page 15. The leaves steeped in vinegar and water will soothe inflammations, painful skin conditions, and hemorrhoids when used externally as a poultice. They may be used in tincture form, fifteen to forty drops every two to four hours.

Homeopathic Uses: Homeopaths use the oil of mullein flowers for earaches. Just cover the flowers in good olive oil and steep them in a closed container in the hot sun for twenty-one days. Strain out the flowers and place the oil directly in the ear. Pack with cotton.

Magical Uses: Known as "hag's tapers," the old stems of mullein were once soaked in fat or wax and used as torches. In ancient grimoires (handbooks of spells) the powdered leaf is a substitute for graveyard dust.

NIGHTSHADE, *SOLANUM DULCAMARA*

Parts Used: Bark of root, and twig.

Herbal Uses: Make nightshade into a salve with chamomile for swellings, bruises, and sprains. In a salve with yellow dock, it treats skin diseases and sores. Make the salve by covering the herbs with olive oil and simmering them for twenty minutes. In a separate pot, bring three or four tablespoons of natural beeswax to a simmer for every cup of olive oil used. When the oil and the wax are the same temperature, combine them, strain, and bottle.
    CAUTION: *This plant is poisonous! Not for internal use.*

Homeopathic Uses: Homeopaths use *Solanum nigrum* (the black nightshade) for violent headaches, convulsions, and meningitis.

Magical Uses: Nightshade placed somewhere on the body will dispel the memory of old loves and protect against evil influences.

PUMPKIN, *CUCURBITA PEPO*

Part Used: Seed.

Herbal Uses: Pumpkin is a New World plant that has recently entered the neo-Pagan tradition. The seed is useful against worms. Make "pumpkin milk" by blending the seeds with water; use seven to fourteen ounces of seed for a child, up to twenty-five ounces for an adult. Drink on an empty stomach, and follow three hours later with a dose of castor oil. In cases of tapeworm, be sure the entire worm is expelled (repeat the dose if needed). The roasted or raw seeds are said to strengthen the male reproductive organ and can be eaten freely.

Homeopathic Uses: Homeopaths use a tincture of the pumpkin seed for nausea of pregnancy and seasickness.

Magical Uses: To the ancient Celts, the spirit of a person was located in the head. Light a candle in your jack-o'-lantern to honor the spirits of the living and the dead.

SAGE, *SALVIA OFFICINALIS*

Part Used: Leaf.

Herbal Uses: Sage is a drying agent for the body. The tea of the leaf will dry up night sweats, breast milk, and mucous congestion. It benefits the nerves and the menstrual cycle as well. Being astringent, it helps with diarrhea. Use it as a sore throat gargle and as a poultice for sores and stings. Use two teaspoons of the herb per cup of water, steep for twenty minutes and take a quarter cup four times a day. Tincture: fifteen to forty drops, up to four times a day.

Homeopathic Uses: Homeopaths use sage for night sweats, coughs, and to dry breast milk.

Magical Uses: Tradition holds that those who eat sage become immortal both in wisdom and in years. Sage is used in wish manifestation and to attract money.

TURNIP, *BRASSICA RAPA*

Parts Used: Seed and root.

Herbal Uses: Turnip root is used in salves and poultices for chilblains; follow the general directions for salves and poultices in chapter 2, "Herbal Basics." The seed helps diarrhea, wet coughs, sneezing, and abdominal fullness caused by incomplete digestion; use six to twelve grams in tea or capsules. Radish seeds (*Raphanus sativus*) have similar properties. The root, when eaten, is said to improve the body's resistance to stress and disease.

> **CAUTION:** *Turnip seed is contraindicated for those who are very weak.*

Magical Uses: Turnips can be hollowed out and a candle placed inside at Samhain. Place them in windows to protect the house from any evil or harm.

WORMWOOD, *ARTEMISIA ABSINTHIUM*

Parts Used: Leaf and flower.

Herbal Uses: The leaves and flowers are used in a light infusion to help digestion, flatulence, and heartburn. Wormwood improves circulation and stimulates the liver. The tea is said to help relieve labor pains. Use one teaspoon per cup and steep for twenty minutes; take a quarter cup up to four times a day; or use as a tincture, eight to ten drops in water up to three times a day. A fomentation of the leaves and flowers soothes bruises and sprains. The oil relieves arthritis.

> **CAUTION:** *The oil is for external use only! Prolonged use of wormwood can lead to nerve damage.*

Homeopathic Uses: Homeopaths use wormwood for epilepsy, insomnia, tremors, and vertigo, especially when accompanied by nausea and bloating.

Magical Uses: The scent of wormwood is said to increase psychic powers. Burned in the graveyard, it is used to summon the spirits of the departed.

CHAPTER 4

Meán Geimhridh
Winter Solstice, Yule

Cold, cold!
Cold tonight is broad Moylurg
Higher the snow than the mountain-range,
The deer cannot get at their food.

from Dillon, **Early Irish Literature**

Cold till Doom!
The storm has spread over all:
A river is each furrow upon the slope,
Each ford a full pool.

from Dillon, **Early Irish Literature**

At Meán Geimhridh, the dark force, with which the Sun battles all winter, gives way. The first rays of light pierce the hollow dark in preparation for the gestation of the seeds that lie fallow under the blanket of the coldest season.

Bonfires are lit in the fields, and crops and trees are "wassailed" loudly with toasts of cider. After a feast, the company repairs to the barn, where the family herd is toasted and a plum cake is hung on a horn of one of the oxen. The beast is doused with cider until he throws off the cake. If it lands in front of him, a bountiful harvest is assured for the coming year.*

---

* Some "Yule" customs listed here are actually Germanic and were adopted by Celtic communities relatively recently.

The Yule log is ceremonially burned in the central fireplace of the home. It must come from a tree on the householder's land or as a gift from a friend; it must never be bought. The log is dragged to the house, decorated with greenery, and doused in cider or ale. Corn or wheat flour is sprinkled on the wood before it is lit.

The Yule log is kindled with a piece from last year's fire and allowed to smolder for twelve days before it is ceremonially put out. Oak, ash, or beech is a good choice for its wood. The ashes are mixed in with the herd animals' water, and an unburned portion is attached to the plow to bless the earth. Ashes are carefully preserved to be mixed with seed for spring plantings. In this way, the sun's power and radiance, symbolically embodied in the burning wood, are spread throughout the land.

Children are escorted to neighbors' homes bearing clove-studded apples and oranges, laid in baskets of evergreens and wheat stalks and dusted with flour. The apples represent the sun, the source of all life. The evergreens are symbols of immortality. The stalks of wheat represent the harvest—the triumph of the forces of light and life.

Holly, ivy, mistletoe, and other greens decorate the house. A house so decorated is prepared to welcome the nature spirits who may be seeking safe shelter from the cold and dark outside. A sprig of holly is retained all year for good luck.

The deities honored at Meán Geimhridh are the Dagda (see chapter 3, "Samhain," for the personification of In Dagda) and Brighid, daughter of the Dagda, patroness of the Druids and Bards, and Goddess of healing, smithcraft, music, and poetry.

Brighid is the patroness of craftsmen, artists of all kinds, and stock animals. She is especially associated with pure white bulls. To understand the connection, we must examine the mysteries of the Egyptian Hathor, the Queen of Heaven, whose symbol is a cow with the solar disk between its horns. The horns are said to represent the physical portal of the human female through which the child emerges, as well as the gateway to spiritual rebirth. The horns also represent the descent of spiritual light into matter (*mater*, Mother) in the great cauldron of the womb. Through the transforming power of the Goddess, the initiate reconnects with her spiritual source.

It is known that the Druids sometimes wore a bull's hide (along with a headdress with a white speckled bird's wings), and that one bardic initiation consisted of being sewn into a leather bag for three days and nights.

Some believe that Brighid was once known as the Great Goddess, the

Creatrix and All-Mother. Today she is remembered as Saint Brighid (or Saint Bride) of Kildare and as such is venerated at holy wells, churches, and shrines. "Kildare" comes from the Gaelic "Cill Dara," "Church of the Oak." According to tradition, Saint Bride was born at dawn, and a column of flame was seen to reach from her head to the highest heavens. Saint Bride is the patroness of childbirth and according to legend was midwife to the Virgin Mary. Fire had always been sacred to the Goddess Brighid. During the ninth century, Irish nuns kept a perpetual fire burning at her shrine in Kildare. Their activities were cut off during the reign of Henry VIII, at the time of the dispossession of the monasteries.

The Iníonacha an Daghdha (the Dagda's daughters) were nine women who tended the sacred fire shrine at Kildare until the office was taken over by Saint Brighid's nuns. These nine would receive Brighid's inspirations and share them with the village women. They excelled in herbcraft and the lore of the healing springs. Brighid's wells were known to cure barrenness and leprosy.

Brighid enlightened the smiths, teaching them the arts of fire tending and the secrets of metalworking. From her came inspired legends, poetry, and music to the bards. Brighid's flame of inspiration, like the flame of winter's new light, pierces the darkness of the mind and spirit at Yuletide, while the cauldron of the Dagda brings assurance that Nature will continue to provide for all of his children.

THE HERBS OF MEÁN GEIMHRIDH

Arborvitae (Yellow Cedar), Ash, Bay Laurel, Blessed Thistle, Chamomile, Frankincense, Holly, Juniper, Mistletoe, Pine

---

Bring some fresh evergreens into the house as a sign to woodland spirits that they may find safe refuge in your home.

Please refer to chapter 2, "Herbal Basics," for methods of preparation.

ARBORVITAE (YELLOW CEDAR), *THUJA OCCIDENTALIS*

Parts Used and Herbal Uses: Please see page 25 in "The Herbs of Samhain."

Magical Uses: Cedar smoke purifies the home. Use it in smudge sticks, incense, and sweat lodges. The scent is said to enhance psychic powers.

ASH, *FRAXINUS EXCELSIOR, FRAXINUS AMERICANA*

Parts Used: Bark and leaf.

Herbal Uses: The bark of the ash can be used as a substitute for quinine in intermittent fevers. It is reputed to clear obstructions from the spleen and liver. Simmer two tablespoons of bark for twenty minutes in one cup of water; take a quarter cup four times a day. The leaves are laxative and can be used as a substitute for senna (tree leaves are always gathered *before* midsummer). Steep two tablespoons of the leaf in one cup of water for twenty minutes; take a quarter cup a day.

Homeopathic Uses: Homeopaths use *Fraxinus americana* for uterine tumors and fibroids. *Fraxinus excelsior* is used for gout and rheumatism.

Magical Uses: Ash is the sacred world tree of the Teutons, known as Yggdrasil. Healing wands and protective staffs are made of ash. Ash wood makes a traditional Yule log. An herb of the sun, ash brings light into the hearth at the winter solstice.

BAY LAUREL, *LAURUS NOBILIS*

Parts Used: Leaf and berry.

Herbal Uses: The leaf and berry are used in salves for itching, sprains, bruises, skin irritations, and rheumatic pain (follow the general directions for salves on page 14). The fruit and leaf are simmered until soft and made into a poultice with honey for chest colds (follow the general directions for poultices on page 15). Bay leaf and berry tea makes a bath additive that helps the bladder, bowel, and female reproductive organs. Use two tablespoons per cup and steep for forty-five minutes; add to bath water.

Magical Uses: Bay leaves were used by the Delphic priestesses. The incense and the leaf are said to induce a prophetic trance. An herb of the sun, bay brings the light of summer into the darkest time of the year. Carry the leaf or place it in the home to ward off illness and hexes.

BLESSED THISTLE, *CARDUUS BENEDICTUS, CNICUS BENEDICTUS, CARBENIA BENEDICTA*

Parts Used: Leaf and stem.

Herbal Uses: Blessed thistle was known to the ancients as a liver tonic. It strengthens the memory, helps with depression, and is useful in migraine headache. Combine it with peppermint, elder flowers, and ginger for colds, fevers, and backache. Blessed thistle is used to promote breast milk (the leaf is the part used). It can be eaten raw in sandwiches and salads, or taken powdered in wine or tea. Use two teaspoons per cup and steep for twenty minutes; take a quarter cup four times a day.

Homeopathic Uses: Homeopaths use *Carduus benedictus* for nausea, left-sided stomach pain, gallstones, surging of blood, homesickness, intermittent fever, and enlarged liver, especially when eye symptoms are present and there is a sensation of contraction in many parts.

Magical Uses: Blessed thistle is an herb of protection used in the ritual bath. It is also used to counteract hexing. Thistle brings spiritual, physical, and financial blessings. Carry one to bring joy, energy, vitality, and protection. A shirt with thistle fibers woven into it will protect the wearer from any evil spell. Thistles make men better lovers. The herb has been used to make magical wands and to conjure or communicate with spirits.

CHAMOMILE, *ANTHEMIS NOBILIS, MATRICARIA CHAMOMILLA*

Part Used: Flower.

Herbal Uses: This herb has an affinity for the solar plexus area of the human body. Colic, upset stomachs, and fevers are benefited by the tea of the fresh or dried flower. Use two tablespoons per cup, steep for twenty minutes, and take a quarter cup four times a day. Women with menstrual cramps can try adding a few thin slices of fresh ginger root to the tea. Chamomile is an antibacterial. Sores, wounds, itches, and rashes respond to external applications. Use the tea as a wash or add the herb to salves and poultices; follow the general directions for salves and poultices on pages 14 and 15. The oil is rubbed into swollen joints. Chamomile calms the nerves and brings on sleep. Use it in baths and gargles. Add the tea to a vaporizer to help asthmatic children. The classic tea for cranky, teething babies, it is given in the bottle or through a mother's breast milk.

Homeopathic Uses: Homeopaths use *Chamomilla* (German chamomile) for earaches and other childhood conditions, especially when the child is whiny, irritable, snappish, thirsty, hot, or restless.

Magical Uses: Yellow chamomile brings the power of the sun to love potions, money spells, and rites of purification. Sprinkle it around the house to ward off hexes.

FRANKINCENSE (OLIBANUM), *BOSWELLIA THURIFERA, BOSWELLIA CARTERII*

Part Used: Resin.

Herbal Uses: A tree resin from southern Arabia, according to Pliny it is an antidote to hemlock poisoning. Avicenna advocated its use for tumors, fevers, vomiting, and dysentery. Chinese herbalists use it in powder form and in teas for rheumatism and menstrual pain, and externally as a wash for sores and bruises. The dose is three to six grains in a glass of wine; or twenty drops of the tincture. Frankincense is highly antiseptic, and the scent is said to calm and clear the mind.
   CAUTION: *Prolonged use of resins can damage the kidneys.*

Magical Uses: Sacred to the Sun God Ra, frankincense is burned in rites of exorcism, purification, and protection. It is said to accelerate spiritual growth. Rosemary may be used as a substitute.

HOLLY (ENGLISH HOLLY), *ILEX AQUIFOLIUM*

Part Used: Leaf.

Herbal Uses: The leaf is dried and used as tea for fevers, bronchitis, bladder problems, and gout. Steep a half ounce of the chopped leaf in boiled water for twenty minutes; take up to one cup a day. The juice of the fresh leaf is helpful in jaundice; take one tablespoon per day. This is the familiar holly of Christmas decorations.
   CAUTION: *The berries are poisonous.*

Homeopathic Uses: Holly can be used as a substitute for quinine. Homeopaths use *Ilex aquifolium* for intermittent fevers, spleen pain, and eye symptoms, especially when the symptoms are better in winter.

Magical Uses: Holly, with its warrior-like bristles, is known as an herb of protection. Cast it about to repel unwanted animals and spirits. Sprinkle newborn babies with "holly water" (water in which holly has been soaked, especially if left under a full moon overnight) to keep them happy and safe. Holly is one of the evergreens brought into the home by Druids. It symbolizes a willingness to allow the nature spirits to share one's abode during the harsh, cold season.

JUNIPER, *JUNIPERUS COMMUNIS*

Parts Used: Berry and young twig.

Herbal Uses: Primarily a diuretic, the berries help digestive problems, gastrointestinal inflammations, and rheumatism. The berries are taken as a tea (simmer two teaspoons per cup for ten minutes; take up to one cup four times a day), or taken as jam or syrup in water, milk, or herb tea. The dry berries can be chewed; three a day is sufficient.

   CAUTION: *Pregnant women and people with weak kidneys should not use juniper berry.*

Homeopathic Uses: Homeopaths use *Juniperus communis* for kidney inflammations, edema with suppressed urine, and faulty digestion. Bloody urine with a cough may be an indication for this remedy as well.

Magical Uses: Juniper when burned is a purifying and protective herb. Men use the berries to increase potency. The herb enhances psychic powers and attracts love.

MISTLETOE, *VISCUM ALBUM*

Parts Used: Twig and leaf.

Herbal Uses: Please see page 100 in "The Herbs of the Druids."

Magical Uses: Mistletoe is gathered at Midsummer or at the sixth day of the moon. Mistletoe will aid and strengthen all magical workings but is perhaps best called upon for healing, protection, and beautiful dreams. It is traditionally hung in the home at Yule, and those who walk under it exchange a kiss of peace.

PINE, *PINUS* SPP.

Parts Used: Needle, twig, and knot of the wood.

Herbal Uses: The needles and young twigs of the white pine (*Pinus strobus, Pinus alba*) are made into infusions for coughs and as an anti-scorbutic; use two teaspoons per cup of water and simmer for twenty minutes. High in vitamin C, they helped our ancestors get through the long winters. The knot of the wood is boiled with angelica, acanthopanax, quince, and mulberry branches to make a bath for arthritis and rheumatism. Pine needles are simmered into massage oils. The oil is used externally to relieve rheumatic pain, chronic bronchitis, sciatica, pneumonia, and nephritis. Simply cover the needles with a good quality olive oil and simmer at a low heat for twenty minutes or place in a low (180°) oven overnight. The resin heals the kidneys, liver, and lungs. The scent is calming to the lungs and nerves.

Homeopathic Uses: Homeopaths use *Pinus sylvestris* (Scotch pine) for rheumatism with bronchial symptoms and an itchy rash. Hemlock (*Tsuga canadensis = Pinus canadensis = Abies canadensis*) is indicated for gnawing hunger, fever, and chills. *Picea mariana = Abies nigra* (Black Spruce) is used for stomach pains that come after eating, after drinking tea or using tobacco, and in the aged, who experience constipation and heart symptoms.

Magical Uses: Pine is the "tree of peace" of the Native American Iroquois confederacy. Burn pine to purify the home, and decorate with its branches to bring healing and joy. Pine needles when burned are said to send spells back to the sender.

CHAPTER 5

Imbolc/Oimealg

Candlemas

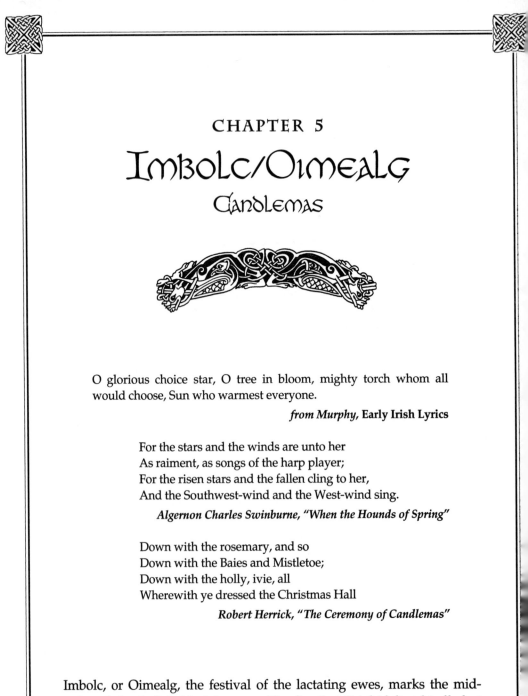

O glorious choice star, O tree in bloom, mighty torch whom all would choose, Sun who warmest everyone.

from Murphy, **Early Irish Lyrics**

> For the stars and the winds are unto her
> As raiment, as songs of the harp player;
> For the risen stars and the fallen cling to her,
> And the Southwest-wind and the West-wind sing.
>
> *Algernon Charles Swinburne, "When the Hounds of Spring"*

> Down with the rosemary, and so
> Down with the Baies and Mistletoe;
> Down with the holly, ivie, all
> Wherewith ye dressed the Christmas Hall
>
> *Robert Herrick, "The Ceremony of Candlemas"*

Imbolc, or Oimealg, the festival of the lactating ewes, marks the midpoint of the dark half of the year. The fire that Brighid first kindled at Yule burns bright in the swollen bellies of pregnant herd animals, and rivers of milk begin to flow in swollen teats and udders.

Agricultural tools are consecrated for the work of the year ahead, household fires are put out and relit, and the fires of the smithy are blessed by a woman acting on Brighid's behalf.

"Brighid's crosses," woven of wheat, are made and given as protective charms for the home. Brighid's snake emerges from the womb of the Earth Mother to test the weather (this is the origin of Ground Hog Day). Even the climate seems to mark the festival; the first week of February typically brings a temporary thaw.

Straw *brideóga* (corn dollies) are fashioned from oat straw or wheat, and dressed and carried door to door by young girls on Imbolc Eve. Each household bestows a small present on the image of the "bride."

Special cakes are baked for the occasion, and a feast and a dance are held for all. The older women of the community gather "bride's beds," or cradles for the corn dollies to sleep in, and magic wands for the dolls to hold. The morning after the feast, everyone examines the ashes of the hearth to see if a magic wand has left marks. If so, it is a good omen for the following year.

In some areas, Imbolc marks the first official day of ploughing, and a decorated plough is dragged from door to door. Children in costumes follow the plough and ask for gifts of food, money, or drink at every home. Any household that refuses them is paid back by having its front garden ploughed up.

The plough itself is a significant symbol of the Imbolc ceremonies. Whiskey, the "water of life," is poured over the blade, or pieces of bread and cheese are left on it to become food for nature spirits. Offerings of food or drink are placed in the new furrows or thrown into the fields.

While Imbolc is principally associated with Brighid, Aengus Og is the male aspect of deity who appears here in the calendar of the ritual year. Son of the Dagda, he is the Celtic version of Eros and the embodiment of youthful love.

Aengus was sick with love for Caer Ibormeith (Yew Berry), and went with Badbh to Loch Bel Dracon to find her. At the lake, they met one hundred and fifty grown women, who were bound to each other with chains of silver. Caer Ibormeith, the tallest, wore a silver choker with a golden chain.

Aillill, the king of Connacht, went to Caer Ibormeith's father to try to win her for Aengus. Her father refused him on the grounds that Caer's magic was stronger than his: Caer, a shape-changer, lived as swan and maiden in alternate years.

At the next feast of Samhain, Caer and her women were scheduled to transform themselves into birds. The only hope that Aengus had of winning her was to take her at this time when she was most vulnerable. Aengus, in human form, called to the swan-maiden Caer, and at that moment he also became a swan. Together, they took to the skies singing magical music that put to sleep for three days and three nights everyone who heard it. Aengus then escorted Caer to her Otherworldly home.

Imbolc is the festival of new beginnings: first ploughing, first planting, and the first fires of new romance. It is the great festival of the milk of the Mother who feeds her children with the fires of life and love.

THE HERBS OF IMBOLC/OIMEALG

Angelica, Basil, Bay, Benzoin, Blackberry, Celandine,
Coltsfoot, Heather, Iris, Myrrh, Tansy, Violets

Burn the greens you brought into the house at winter solstice.
Please refer to chapter 2, "Herbal Basics," for methods of preparation.

ANGELICA, *ANGELICA ARCHANGELICA*

Part Used: Root.

Herbal Uses: Used in infusion or tincture, the root raises body temperature and promotes digestion, making it an ideal herb for older folks. It also helps bring down the menses. Use it for colds and flu, to induce a sweat and warm the body. The decoction of the dried root is said to remove the taste for alcohol. Simmer two teaspoons of the root in two cups of water for twenty minutes; take one cup twice a day.

Use the root in salves for skin problems and rheumatic pains (follow the general directions for salves on page 14). The tincture can be used in doses of ten to thirty drops, four times a day.

CAUTION: *Do not exceed the indicated amounts, or the heart, blood pressure, and respiration can be affected.*

Magical Uses: Angelica leaves are scattered to purify an area. Add them to incense to promote healing. The leaves can be smoked in herbal "tobacco" formulas.

BASIL, *Ocimum basilicum*

Parts Used: Leaf and stem.

Herbal Uses: The infusion relieves gas and stomach pains. Reputedly abortive, it can help expel the placenta. A warming herb, it is used for colds and flu, constipation, vomiting, headaches, and menstrual cramps. Steep two teaspoons per cup of water for twenty minutes; take up to one and a half cups per day.

Magical Uses: Basil is used to mend lovers' quarrels and in love spells. Basil attracts money and brings good luck to a new home. Use it in rites of exorcism and in the ritual bath. Sprinkle the powder over the area of your heart to promote fidelity. The scent brings happiness to the home and will protect you in crowds.

BAY LAUREL, *Laurus nobilis*

Parts Used and Herbal Uses: Please see page 33 in "The Herbs of Meán Geimhridh."

Magical Uses: Bay is burned to induce trances. An herb of the sun, it brings light and purification to the home when burned.

BLACKBERRY, *Rubus villosus*

Parts Used: Root, leaf, bud, and berry.

Herbal Uses: The root is a classic remedy for diarrhea and is reputed to clean the kidneys and urinary tract of stones and gravel. Simmer two teaspoons of the root per cup of water for twenty minutes, and take a quarter cup four times a day. The buds and leaves are used fresh in poultices for wounds, burns, mouth sores, and sore throats. Chew the leaves or follow the general directions for poultices on page 15. The berries are slightly binding (as is blackberry wine) and are useful in diarrhea, as are the leaves.

Homeopathic Uses: Homeopaths use *Rubus villosus* for diarrhea of infancy, with watery and clay-colored stool.

Magical Uses: Sacred to Brighid, the leaves and berries are used to attract wealth or healing. This is a Goddess herb, belonging to the planetary sphere of Venus.

CELANDINE, *CHELIDONIUM MAJUS*

Parts Used: Leaf, stem, and root.

Herbal Uses: **CAUTION:** *Some people are sensitive to this plant and may experience skin irritation when picking it.* The dried plant is less irritating. This herb is *powerful* and should be taken only once to bring about its effects. Internally, the tincture or infusion of the leaf will stimulate and clean the liver. To make tea, simmer one teaspoon herb or root in one cup boiled water for thirty minutes; it will boil down to one-half cup. Drink this tea cold, sipping it through the day. For tincture, the dose is ten to fifteen drops. Jaundice, and complaints of the gallbladder, liver, and stomach are benefited by this plant. Externally, the salve has been used to clear eczema, scrofula, and herpes; follow the general directions for salve on page 14. The fresh juice is dabbed two or three times a day on warts, ringworm, and corns.

   CAUTION: *Do not allow it to touch other parts of the skin.*

Homeopathic Uses: Homeopaths use *Chelidonium majus* for jaundice with pain under the right scapula. Icy coldness of fingertips and alternating diarrhea and constipation are indications, as is a loose cough with right-sided chest pain. These ailments are worse with changes of weather.

Magical Uses: Celandine brings joy and cures depression. Wear it to escape entrapments and as a protective herb.

COLTSFOOT, *TUSSILAGO FARFARA*

Parts Used: Leaf and flower.

Herbal Uses: The yellow flowers of coltsfoot resemble the sun, and it is among the first plants to emerge in the spring, often when snow remains on the ground. The leaves appear after the flowers have bloomed. This plant, once called British tobacco, can be smoked to relieve coughs and shortness of breath. The tea is useful for all lung, sinus, and throat conditions and for diarrhea. Steep two teaspoons of leaf per cup of water for twenty minutes. Coltsfoot is applied as a poultice to stings, swellings, burns, ulcers, and phlebitis (follow the general directions for poultices on page 15).

Homeopathic Uses: Homeopaths use coltsfoot as an intercurrent remedy in pneumonia.

Magical Uses: "Sponnc" (the Gaelic for coltsfoot) is an herb sacred to Brighid. Coltsfoot, an herb of Venus, is used magically to engender love and to bring peace.

HEATHER, *CALLUNA VULGARIS*

Part Used: Flowering shoot.

Herbal Uses: The flowering shoots of heather are used for insomnia, stomach pains, coughs, and skin problems. Heather, used fresh or dry, strengthens the heart and slightly raises the blood pressure. Heather is slightly diuretic. Fresh or dried heather shoots are simmered, four teaspoons to the cup; the dose is one-half cup per day.

Magical Uses: White heather brings good luck and protects the one who wears it. Dip heather and fern in water and sprinkle around to conjure rain. Heather is a Goddess herb associated with the planet Venus and sacred to Isis.

IRIS (BLUE FLAG), *IRIS VERSICOLOR*

Parts Used: Root and leaf.

Herbal Uses: Iris root is found in the swamps of North America. Just as iris purifies the mud of boggy areas, so does it clean the human bowel. Chronic liver problems and digestive problems will benefit from this plant, as will nonmalignant enlargements of the thyroid. Stomach-centered migraine headaches and chronic sinus congestion are helped by it. Iris is taken in tincture, ten to twenty-five drops in water, three times a day. The fresh leaf is used in poultices for burns and injuries. The root is gathered in the fall and taken as a decoction for colds. Simmer one teaspoon per pint of water for twenty minutes; take three tablespoons six times a day, cold.

 CAUTION: *The fresh root causes skin irritation in some individuals.*

Homeopathic Uses: Homeopaths use *Iris versicolor* for frontal headaches with nausea, constipation, ringing in the ears, psoriasis, eczema, and rheumatism. The pancreas and gastrointestinal tract are a strong focus for this remedy, especially when symptoms worsen after sundown or after resting.

Magical Uses: The fresh flowers are said to purify an area and to attract the qualities of wisdom, faith, and courage. Sacred to Iris, Goddess of the Rainbow, to Juno, and to the sphere of Venus, iris is a classic Goddess herb.

MYRRH, *COMMIPHORA MYRRHA*

Parts Used: Resin.

Herbal Uses: Especially valued as a disinfectant, myrrh, a tree resin, is used as a wash for wounds. CAUTION: *Use as a wound wash only after the wound has been well cleaned.* It has the tendency to seal wounds once it is placed on them. Use the alcohol tincture in water or the tea as a wound wash. Myrrh promotes circulation and increases heart rate and power. Said to move stagnant blood through the uterus, it has been used for menopause, menstrual irregularities, and uterine tumors. Myrrh benefits diabetes and obesity; the dose is one to fifteen grains. Combined with echinacea and mullein, the tea helps ear infections. Use equal parts of echinacea and mullein to one quarter part myrrh; steep two teaspoons per cup of water for twenty minutes; take a quarter cup every four hours. (Try packing the ear with cotton soaked in mullein oil as well—see page 27 in "The Herbs of Samhain.") Myrrh, goldenseal, arnica, and cayenne can be soaked in rubbing alcohol for a few weeks to make a liniment for bruises and sprains.

CAUTION: *Prolonged internal use of myrrh (longer than a few weeks) could lead to kidney damage.*

Magical Uses: Myrrh is a Goddess plant of the Moon's sphere, sacred to Isis. Burned, it brings peace, healing, consecration, and blessing. Myrrh aids contemplation and meditation.

TANSY, *TANACETUM VULGARE*

Part Used: Flower head.

Herbal Uses: The infusion of dried tansy leaves and flowers is taken while one is fasting to expel worms; steep one teaspoon per cup for twenty minutes, and take one cup on an empty stomach night and morning. Taken three times a day, it helps induce menstruation. The leaf is said to be a tonic for the heart. (Infuse one fresh leaf a day in herb tea.) Tansy is a good remedy for worms in children. The flowers and seeds are helpful for gout. Tansy and elderleaf make a natural insecticide when boiled and sprayed on plants.

CAUTION: *Pregnant women should avoid tansy as it has been shown to be abortive in large doses.*

Homeopathic Uses: Homeopaths use *Tanacetum vulgare* for poison ivy, abnormal lassitude, and worms. Dysentery, suppressed menstruation, labored breath, and a sensation as if the ears were roaring, ringing, and "closed up suddenly" are symptoms addressed by this herb.

Magical Uses: Once used to preserve dead bodies, tansy is known as an herb of immortality and longevity.

VIOLET, *VIOLA ODORATA*

Part Used: Whole plant.

Herbal Uses: The whole plant is used, fresh or dry. The leaves can be eaten as a type of wild spinach, and the flowers are used in salads and desserts. High in iron, the fresh leaf is used internally and externally for cancer, especially of the colon, throat, and tongue. For this purpose, the fresh leaves should be infused daily and taken as tea; using one teaspoon of plant parts to a half cup of water, steep and take a quarter cup four times a day. The tea can be applied externally as a fomentation. The flowers are laxative; the roots and stems are emetic and purgative. The fresh leaves are used in salves and poultices for wounds; follow the general directions for salves and poultices on pages 14 and 15.

Homeopathic Uses: Homeopaths use *Viola odorata* for right-sided complaints, especially burning of the forehead, tension of the scalp and ears, headache across the forehead, discharge from the ears, labored breathing during pregnancy, milky urine, and pressing pain in the joints of the wrist and hand.

Magical Uses: Violet crowns are said to cure headache, bring sleep, and calm anger. Violets are mixed with lavender, apple blossoms, yarrow, and roses in love potions. The leaf is a protection from all evil.

CHAPTER 6

Meán Earraigh

Spring Equinox

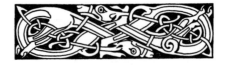

And frosts are slain and flowers begotten,
And in green underworld and cover
Blossom by blossom the spring begins.

Algernon Charles Swinburne,
"When the Hounds of Spring"

wholly to be a fool
while Spring is in the world

my blood approves

e. e. cummings, "since feeling is first"

Meán Earraigh marks the spring equinox, when night and day are of equal length and spring officially begins. Birds begin their nesting and egg-laying, and eggs—symbolic of rebirth, fertility, and immortality—are tossed into fresh furrows or eaten by ploughmen. They are also carried by those engaged in spring planting.

A charming custom is painting eggs with symbols and pictures of what one wishes to manifest in the coming year. The eggs can then be buried in the Earth Mother, who hears the cries and dreams of her children.

In some communities, eggs are hidden in the stores of seed grain and left there all season to bless the sowing and encourage the seeds to sprout. Dressed as mummers, "pace-eggers" go from house to house and demand eggs and coins in return for a short performance. Men and women exchange clothing for the show.

The eggs given to the pace-eggers have been wrapped in leaves, roots, flowers, and bark before boiling, to impart color. Later, the eggs are used in games, such as attempting to strike an opponent's legs. The eggs might be hidden or rolled down hillsides, after which they are eaten.

Blood, ashes from sacred fires, fistfuls of salt, or handfuls of soil from a high mountaintop are scattered on the newly sown fields. Offerings of food and milk are left for the fairies and other spirits who live in and around rocks and are responsible for the fertility of the land. A few fruits from the previous year's harvest are left for the nature spirits.

Sacred hilltops are visited, and picnics of figs, fig cakes, cider, and ale are enjoyed. The figs are symbolic of fertility, the leaf being the male element and the fruit the female.

Aengus Og is the male deity of the occasion. Son of In Dagda and Boand, he was conceived and born while Elcmar, Boand's husband, was under enchantment. When three days old, Aengus was removed to be fostered by Midir, god of the Otherworld mound at Bri Leith, with his three hostile cranes. These birds guarded the mound and prevented the approach of travelers, and were said to cause even warriors to turn and flee.

Aengus, Son of the Dawn, and In Dagda are the deities associated with Newgrange (Bruig na Boinne), the great solar temple in the Boyne Valley of Ireland. While the Dagda plays a harp of oak, Aengus plays his harp of gold to the young and blows kisses, which engender amorous desires.

The female aspect of this festival is personified by Boand herself, who is sometimes equated with the River Boyne. A legend claims that the Boyne sprang into being when the Goddess Boand was disrespectful of the magical well of Segais. The well rose in anger, the goddess fled, and the River Boyne was created.

Boand is known as "She of the White Cows." It is worthwhile to remember that Brighid was raised on the milk of a white cow with red ears. Otherworldly beasts such as dogs and cows are generally described with this coloring. Sacred kine are often said to emerge from lakes; water is the entrance to the Otherworld.

If you visit the River Boyne, you will find that she is quite maternal, flowing gently and sweetly and giving of herself to the land—like a placid milk cow.

The Herbs of Meán Earraigh

Acorn, Celandine, Cinquefoil, Dandelion, Dogwood,
Honeysuckle (Woodbine), Iris, Jasmine, Rose, Tansy, Violet.

Plant some spring flowers. Bless some seeds for the garden.
Please refer to chapter 2, "Herbal Basics," for methods of preparation.

Acorn, Quercus spp.

Parts Used and Herbal Uses: Please see page 23 in "The Herbs of Samhain."

Magical Uses: Acorns bring fertility and luck to all projects.

Celandine, Chelidonium majus

Parts Used and Herbal Uses: Please see page 42 in "The Herbs of Imbolc/ Oimealg."

Magical Uses: Celandine is an herb of joy and protection.

Cinquefoil, Potentilla reptans, P. canadensis

Parts Used: Root and leaf.

Herbal Uses: The powdered root and the leaf are used to stop internal hemorrhaging. The powder also makes an astringent for mouth sores and relieves diarrhea. Taken with honey, it relieves sore throats, coughs, and fever. Take one-quarter to one-half teaspoon at a time, or twenty to forty drops of the tincture. The leaves can be steeped using two teaspoons per cup for twenty minutes, or one ounce of the root can be simmered in one and a half cups of water for twenty minutes. The dose is a quarter cup four times a day.

Magical Uses: Use the infusion in ritual baths and for purification rites. Cinquefoil bestows eloquence and protection to the wearer; bring it to court. Love, power, wisdom, health, and abundance are symbolized by its five petals. Prick a hole in an egg, drain it, and fill it with cinquefoil. Tape the egg shut, and your home and property are protected. Bathe in the infusion every seven days to ward off evil influences.

DANDELION (WILD ENDIVE), *TARAXACUM OFFICINALE*

Parts Used: Leaf, root, flower.

Herbal Uses: Dandelions love people and will follow us almost into the house if we let them! The leaves are edible in early spring when they are rich in vitamins and iron. Simmer two teaspoons per cup of water for twenty minutes; take three tablespoons six times a day. The root is gathered in fall to make a liver-cleansing tea. The flowers are made into wine.

The fresh juice is the most beneficial part of the plant; one teaspoon three times a day in milk is recommended for constipation, bad digestion, fevers, insomnia, rheumatic conditions, and gout. A dandelion fast in the spring will improve everyone's health. Eat a fresh dandelion leaf salad with olive oil and lemon juice, drink a tea of the chopped root and leaf twice a day, and take several glasses of water with three tablespoons of the juice each day.

Homeopathic Uses: Homeopaths use low potencies of *Taraxacum* for liver-centered headaches, jaundice, cancer of the bladder, gas, night sweats, and neuralgia of the knee. There is a peculiar concomitant, which is a "mapped tongue"—covered with white film and sores, and peeling to leave red, irritated spots. All symptoms become worse when the person is resting, lying down, and sitting.

Magical Uses: Dandelion tea is said to increase psychic abilities, perhaps because of its cleansing and rejuvenating qualities. Simple garden magic: pick a "puff ball" on the night of a full moon, call in the sacred directions, and blow your wish to the winds.

Dandelion belongs to the *Belenountion*: herbs associated with the Celtic Diety Belenos. These are yellow plants that are ritually gathered at midsummer in Brittany. They are said to form the body of the God.

DOGWOOD, *CORNUS FLORIDA*

Parts Used: Dried bark, berry.

Herbal Uses: The dried bark is taken in tincture (20 drops) or tea.

Simmer one tablespoon dried bark per cup for twenty minutes; the dose is a half cup every two or three hours to relieve fevers. It has been used as a substitute for quinine.

A tincture of the berries heals a stomach damaged by alcoholism. Follow the standard directions for tincture on page 15. The dose is twenty drops four times a day. Among some Native American tribes, the flowering of the dogwood signaled the time for corn planting.

Magical Uses: Dogwood leaves, flowers, and wood are a protective charm. The four petals symbolize the sacred four directions and the four elements: Earth, Air, Fire, and Water.

HONEYSUCKLE (WOODBINE), *LONICERA CAPRIFOLIUM*

Part Used: Flower.

Herbal Uses: Properties are cited for the common flower that grows wild, rather than the ornamental varieties. The flowers have a broad-spectrum antimicrobial effect against salmonella, staphyloccus, and streptococcus. Chinese herbalists have long recognized honeysuckle as an antibiotic herb for colds, flus, and fevers. Sore throats, conjunctivitis, and inflammations of the bowel, urinary tract, and reproductive organs have been treated with it. It is said to be useful in treating cancer. Combine it with seeds of *Forsythia suspensii,* the well-known yellow flowering shrub, or *Echinacea augustifolia* or *E. purpurea* for maximum antiviral and antibacterial effect. Steep two teaspoons per cup for twenty minutes. The dose is a quarter cup, four times a day.

Homeopathic Uses: Homeopaths use *Lonicera pericylmenum* for irritability of temper with violent outbursts and *Lonicera xylosteum* for convulsions and coma with a red face, cold temperature, and perspiration.

Magical Uses: Honeysuckle flowers are said to attract money. They will heighten psychic abilities when rubbed on the forehead.

IRIS (BLUE FLAG), *IRIS VERSICOLOR*

Parts Used and Herbal Uses: Please see page 43 in "The Herbs of Imbolc/ Oimealg."

Magical Uses: Iris is a Goddess herb, which brings purity, wisdom, courage, and faith.

JASMINE, *JASMINUM OFFICINALE*

Part Used: Flower.

Herbal Uses: The flowers make a tea that calms the nerves and increases erotic feelings. Steep two teaspoons of flowers per cup of water for twenty minutes. The dose is a quarter cup, four times a day. The oil of the leaf is rubbed on the head to heal the eyes. A syrup of jasmine flowers and honey will help with coughs and lung complaints. The essential oil of jasmine is said to help menstrual pain and lung problems.

> CAUTION: *The berries are poisonous.*

Homeopathic Uses: Homeopaths use a dilute tincture of the berries for tetanus and convulsions. Use only with medical supervision.

Magical Uses: Jasmine flowers will help you attract wealth. The scent is said to bring on prophetic dreams. The flowers are used in love spells to attract a spiritual love.

ROSE, *ROSA* SPP.

Parts Used: Flower and hips.

Herbal Uses: Rose petal syrup can be made by adding twice the petals' weight of sugar and infusing in hot water. Alternatively, the fresh petals can be ground with a little boiling water and strained, and the liquid combined with honey. The resulting liquid is a natural laxative and a tonic for the stomach. The rose hips should be gathered *after* the first frost. They will be red and ready for drying or making into jam. The jam or jelly is used for coughs. The dried hips are opened, the seeds and hairs removed, and the skins used for an excellent sore throat tea; use two teaspoons per cup of water and simmer for ten minutes. An infusion of the petals, one ounce to one pint of water, makes a soothing eye lotion; strain it first through a cheesecloth.

Homeopathic Uses: Homeopaths use *Rosa damascena* (damask rose) for hay fever involving the eustachian tubes, for deafness, and for ringing in the ears.

Magical Uses: Rose buds are added to bath water to conjure a lover. Place some in a red cloth bag and pin it under your clothes. Rose hips worn as beads attract love. Add red rose petals to healing formulas and spells. The rose is a Goddess herb belonging to Venus and the Water element.

TANSY, *TANACETUM VULGARE*

Parts Used and Herbal Uses: Please see page 44 in "The Herbs of Imbolc/Oimealg."

Magical Uses: Tansy is an herb of immortality and longevity.

VIOLET, *VIOLA ODORATA*

Parts Used and Herbal Uses: Please see page 45 in "The Herbs of Imbolc/Oimealg."

Magical Uses: Violets are an herb of love and protection.

CHAPTER 7

Beltaine
May Eve

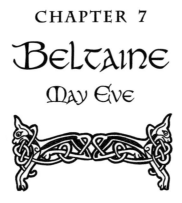

Green bursts out on every herb,
The top of the green oakwood is bushy,
Summer has come, winter has gone
Twisted hollies wound the hound.

The Sun smiles over every land,
A parting for me from the brood of cares:
Hounds bark, stags tryst,
Ravens flourish, summer has come!

from Dillon, **Early Irish Literature**

Beltaine is a profoundly complex festival, with the dual associations of fertility and death. It is on May Eve that the sexual forces of the world are at their peak. The need for balance in nature is also recognized. In ancient times, a life was taken so that the greater life might continue.

Here it is fascinating to reflect on the similarity of the Christian myth with the Druidic. Both recognize the pattern of sacrifice and transcendence as a powerful force for healing in the community.

Beltaine had such deep significance for the Celts that many important historic occasions were said to have taken place on that date. It was at Beltaine that the tribe of Partholon landed on Eire, and they left on the same day three hundred years later. One Beltaine, the Tuatha Dé Danann arrived in Eire; and another Beltaine brought the Sons of Mil.

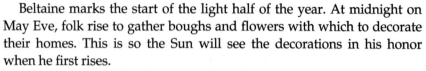

Beltaine marks the start of the light half of the year. At midnight on May Eve, folk rise to gather boughs and flowers with which to decorate their homes. This is so the Sun will see the decorations in his honor when he first rises.

It is the time to offer libations and cakes to the guardian spirits of the flocks and herds, and to the fox, eagle, and crow that they might spare domestic animals.

Young women rise at dawn to bathe their faces in the dew of the hawthorn blossoms and to petition the God or Goddess to give them beauty. Tradition dictates that they wear rowan sprigs as they do this.

Maypoles are erected, the male phallic pole being buried snugly in the female Earth. The pole also represents the movement of energy between Earth and sky that results in the renewal of growth in the spring. Herbs and tree branches are brought into the home as a way of concentrating healing and fertile energies.

Standing stones are visited to ensure a good harvest or abundant rainfall. Rain is invoked by beating the stones with a hazel rod or by throwing water on them. An abundant harvest is achieved by walking three times, sunwise, around a stone and finishing with a bow.

Fisherfolk sprinkle sand at the foot of a stone and walk around it, sunwise, asking for fair weather and a bountiful catch. They may also drop garlands of flowers into the sea to bring good fishing. Flowers and food are offered to stones on the farm or to stones carried to a mountaintop.

Milk is poured into hollows of stones as a gift for the "little people." Ailing children are passed through holes in stones, as are initiates, who are thus symbolically reborn into a new life.

Spiral dances, circle dances, and maypole dances are performed to energize the soil. Young couples disappear into the hills, forests, and newly plowed fields to further energize the land with their activities.

Mock battles are held between a green-and-white-clad "Summer Lord," bedecked with garlands and ribbons, and a fur-clad "Winter Lord" wearing holly. The Summer Lord always wins. Each combatant is carried through the town, bringing the power of the trees and the spirit of the greening grain to all.

Birch wreaths are given as lover's gifts—the traditional maypole was often a birch. But May is an unlucky time for marriage, as the temptations of the season pose a threat to family love and stability. In fact, Beltaine is a traditional time to arrange divorces!

Branches of rowan are placed as protection over the doors of the

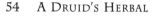

house and barn. Rising at dawn to watch the sunrise from a hilltop is a lucky activity. Apple orchards are visited, and cider and cakes are buried in them.

There is an old tradition of "walking the wheat" whereby a couple or group hold hands and walk across a field, blessing it as they go. Bits of cake are ritually eaten, tossed into the air, and buried to enhance the proceedings.

Fires are kindled in holes in the earth. A "caudle" of butter, oatmeal, eggs, and milk is boiled on the fire. Alcoholic libations are generously added to the brew by everyone. Some of the caudle is ritually poured onto the soil as a libation, and oatmeal cakes are distributed—each with its raised bumps dedicated to some animal or being who is responsible for preserving or harming the herd animals. The caudle is eaten by all, and the remnants are hidden by two designated people, who produce it anew the following Sunday.

"Mayers" go from home to home singing and dancing, and they are given eggs, fruits, cakes, or money for their efforts. These performers bring spring into the village and by their actions encourage generosity and community feeling in the populace. It is hoped that this generosity will be reflected in nature.

A May Queen and King are selected by the celebrants as symbols of the sacred marriage between Earth and Sky. The King is chosen for having won a foot race or having climbed the maypole. Sometimes the Queen is elected by the community and *she* chooses the King. Chimney sweeps are often chosen for this honor. Feasting continues under the maypole, which has been painted with red spirals symbolizing the life force and white spirals symbolizing new beginnings.

Young girls go from home to home carrying a "May Baby," a doll dressed in white and laid in a flower-filled cradle. At each door they sing a song and are given gifts of food or coin.

The element of water is honored in May Day festivities. Dancers construct a "hobby-horse," which wades into a local pond to "drink" and then sprinkle the folk with water. A "May Fool" might carry a pole bedecked with shreds of cloth, resembling a mop, which he dips into a pool to sprinkle all and sundry.

Fire is honored as men leap through the bonfires. Women leap next, and finally the herd animals are driven through the smoking embers as an act of purification and protection. A somewhat related custom is the rolling of a great cheese (a sun symbol) or a burning hoop down a hill.

At every ancient fire festival (Imbolc, Beltaine, Lugnasad, Samhain), the house fires were doused and relit from a sacred central fire managed by Druids. The right to enter and occupy land that had belonged to one's ancestors was the right to uncover the fire. At Uisnach, (the geographic center of Eire and the seat of the archdruid) in the old days, the archdruid lit the great fire from which runners would carry burning torches to all the chief fires of Ireland. (Tlachta in Tara was the site of the central Samhain fire.)

To understand the significance of sacramental fire, we must look at the Vedic tradition, in which Agni is the sacred fire at the center of the Earth. The Pythagoreans believed in a great central fire at the heart of the universe. For Egyptians, the cosmic fire was embodied by the trinity of Ra-Bast-Sekhmet, the Sun, whose great fire was the source of all life.

The darker side of Beltaine is related to the worship of Bile, the Celtic Dis Pater from whom the first people descended. Tradition holds that he sent the first Gaels from the Otherworld to Eire, and in his honor human sacrifices were chosen (or themselves chose) to join him. To accomplish the selection a cake was divided up, with one piece marked by charring. Whoever got the burned piece was the sacrifice.

It is worthwhile to ponder the similarity between this ultimate Druid initiation and the supreme sacrifice of the Christos who, by dying and rising, brought eternal life to his people.

Boand is also honored at the Beltaine feast. It was she who approached the well circled by nine hazel trees. The nuts that fell from the trees had the property of bestowing all knowledge on whoever ate them. Only the divine "Salmon of Knowledge" that lived in the well had permission to swallow the nuts. Even the Gods and Goddesses were forbidden access to the well.

Boand dared to approach the sacred well, but as she did so, the waters rose to drive her away. Thus the River Boyne was born, spreading the blessings of the water and the wisdom of the Salmon throughout the land.

THE HERBS OF BELTAINE

Almond, Belladonna, Clover, Frankincense, Hawthorn, Ivy, Marigold, Meadowsweet, Orchid Root, Rose, Rowan, Sorrel, Woodruff

Plant a flowering tree, and sleep under it with your lover. Leave a May basket on someone's doorstep.

Please refer to chapter 2, "Herbal Basics," for methods of preparation.

ALMOND, *AMYGDALUS COMMUNIS*

Part Used: Nut.

Herbal Uses: Almonds must be chewed well and slowly. The whole raw almond has been described as a cancer preventative. Arabs crossing vast deserts live on only almonds, dates, and water. One ounce of almonds can be soaked overnight in four ounces of water and blended in the morning to make a milk substitute. Peeled almonds can relieve heartburn. Ground almonds make a wonderful facial scrub. The oil relieves coughs and hoarseness. Almonds have very little starch, and the butter and flour of the nuts is recommended for diabetics.

    CAUTION: *Almonds contain hydrocyanic acid and can be toxic if eaten in large amounts (over fifty kernels for an adult, ten for a child).*

Homeopathic Uses: Homeopaths use *Amygdalus amara* (bitter almond) in fresh infusion or as tincture for painful tonsils, difficulty swallowing, vomiting, and a cough with sore chest.

Magical Uses: Magical wands are made of almond wood. In the Greek tradition, Phyllis was deserted by her lover Demophoon and died of grief. The gods changed her into a barren almond tree. When Demophoon returned and embraced the tree, it burst into leaf and flower—a symbol of true love transcending death.

BELLADONNA, *BELLADONA ATROPA*

Parts Used: Leaf, twig, and berry.

Herbal Uses: CAUTION: *This herb is poisonous.* The plant is narcotic and is used for high fevers with attendant inflammation, pain, dilated pupils, and reddened face. The leaves are applied externally as a poultice for cancer. Colitis and kidney pain are relieved by this herb. *One to three drops* of the leaf tincture or *one drop* of the root tincture is the dose.

    CAUTION: *Belladonna can cause paralysis of the central nervous system if overdose occurs. Do not use without medical supervision.*

Homeopathic Uses: Homeopaths use a very dilute preparation of belladonna for conditions showing hot, red skin, flushed face, glaring eyes, throbbing parotid glands, delirium and mental excitement, restless sleep, convulsion, and dryness of mouth and throat with aversion to water (thirstlessness). Violence of attack and suddenness of onset are key indicators. Belladonna is a good remedy for the fevers and ear infections of childhood when characteristic symptoms are present.

Magical Uses: Belladonna is an ingredient of "flying ointments" used traditionally at Walpurgisnacht (May Eve), the traditional celebration of Germanic witches known as Hexen. Flying ointments are preparations of poisonous and psychedelic herbs prepared as a salve. These salves often include soot to help the witch see how much she has put on. When the witch rubs the ointment on the skin, she is enabled to "fly" astrally. Entire covens have been said to fly together in this way to a designated location without actually moving their physical bodies.

CLOVER, *TRIFOLIUM* SPP.

Part Used: Flower.

Herbal Uses: For most uses, the best clover is the red (*T. pratense*), a nutritive plant whose flowers can be eaten in salad, sandwiches, and teas. Red clover is known as a blood and lymph cleanser. Clover tea is mixed with chaparral for cancer therapy. An antitussive, clover calms coughs and promotes expectoration. It is also used for fevers, arthritis, lung inflammation, and gout. Steep two teaspoons of the flowers per cup of water for twenty minutes. The dose is a quarter cup, four times a day. Gather the blossoms while they are fresh and newly opened, and dry them in the shade or tincture them. Follow the standard directions for tinctures on page 15.

Homeopathic Uses: Homeopaths use *Trifolium pratense* (red clover) for conditions characterized by increased flow of saliva, seborrhea with dry scaly crusts, stiff neck, whooping cough, hay fever, and chills. *Trifolium repens* (white clover) is considered a prophylactic against mumps, the symptoms of which include pain and hardness of the submaxillary glands and profuse, watery saliva—all worse when the patient is lying down.

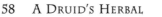

Magical Uses: Clover blossoms are tinctured in vinegar for three days. The vinegar is then sprinkled around the house to discourage unwanted entities. Carry some flowers in your purse or pocket as a protective charm and to attract a new love. Finding a two-leafed clover means a lover will come to you again. The four-leafed clover brings peace of mind, psychic powers, money, and treasure. The five-leafed clover brings money. The white clover counteracts hexes.

FRANKINCENSE (OLIBANUM), *BOSWELLIA THURIFERA, B. CARTERII*

Parts Used and Herbal Uses: Please see page 35 in "The Herbs of Meán Geimhridh."

Magical Uses: Frankincense is an intensely spiritual herb of purification and protection.

HAWTHORN, *CRATAEGUS* SPP.

Parts Used: Berry and flower.

Herbal Uses: The berry is a superior heart tonic, useful for almost any heart condition. Cholesterol problems and valvular diseases are benefited. The berries also strengthen the appetite and digestion. Extended use lowers blood pressure. Hawthorn berry is a good remedy for the nerves and for insomnia. The berries are simmered or tinctured. Simmer two teaspoons of berries per cup of water for twenty minutes. The dose is a quarter cup four times a day. To prepare a tincture, follow the standard instructions for tinctures on page 15. Take ten to twenty drops four times a day. The flowers are taken as tea to benefit the heart. Steep two teaspoons of flowers per cup of water for twenty minutes; the dose is a quarter cup four times a day.

Homeopathic Uses: Homeopaths use hawthorn as a heart tonic for irregular heartbeat, myocarditis, insomnia, edema, arteriosclerosis, and juvenile diabetes.

Magical Uses: Hawthorn is the classic flower to decorate a maypole. An herb of fertility, it finds its place in weddings, May Day celebrations, and ritual groves. Where oak and ash and thorn grow together, one may see fairies. Beltaine was once reckoned as the day the hawthorn first bloomed.

IVY, *HEDERA HELIX*

Parts Used: Twig and leaf.

Herbal Uses: Tender ivy twigs are simmered in salves to heal sunburn; follow the standard instructions for salves on page 14. The leaves are used as a douche for vaginal infections. Externally, ivy is used in poultices to heal nerves, sinews, ulcers, enlarged glands, boils, and abscesses. Follow the standard instructions for poultices on page 15.

Homeopathic Uses: Homeopaths use ivy for conditions with intra-cranial pressure.

Magical Uses: Ivy is equated with fidelity and is woven into marriage wreaths. Use it in charms to bind luck, love, and fidelity to your person.

MARIGOLD, *CALENDULA OFFICINALIS*

Parts Used: Flower and leaf.

Herbal Uses: This is the "pot marigold," not the African variety so common in American gardens. The flowers are a healing agent. Added to fomentations, poultices, and salves, they speed healing of wounds and of nerve damage. Follow the standard instructions for tinctures, poultices, and salves on pages 14 and 15. The infusion is given for intestinal problems and to clean lymph and blood. Useful in fevers, the herb can be used fresh, dry, or in tincture. For tea, steep two teaspoons of flowers per cup of water for twenty minutes; take one teaspoon per hour. Using tincture, take five to twenty drops four times a day.

Homeopathic Uses: Homeopaths use *Calendula officinalis* as a local application to open wounds, to stop bleeding after dental work, and internally for cancer. It is indicated especially for excessive pain and a tendency to be chilled, especially in damp weather.

Magical Uses: Calendula is carried into court for a favorable verdict. In the mattress, it encourages prophetic dreams. Placed under the bed, it can make dreams come true. Added to bath water, it helps attract respect and admiration. Known as "summer's bride," the yellow calendula embodies the Sun's fire and life-sustaining virtue.

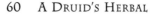

Meadowsweet, *Spiraea ulmaria*

Parts Used and Herbal Uses: Please see page 98 in "The Herbs of the Druids."

Magical Uses: Meadowsweet is used in love spells and is strewn about the home to bring peace and joy.

Orchid Root (Satyrion Root), *Orchis* spp.

Part Used: Root.

Herbal Uses: The root is starchy when gathered in the fall, and is nutritive for children and the bedridden. It is boiled with milk and water and flavored with sassafras, clove, cinnamon, or ginger and a sweetener. One part of the powdered root is mixed with ten parts cold water and then added to ninety parts boiling water to make a soothing demulcent for children's diarrhea and fevers. Salep, the drink made from the roots, was once used to keep sailors alive on long voyages when food was scarce. The root is said to strengthen the genitals and aid in conception.

    Caution: *Most American orchids are rare or endangered. As a rule, wild patches should be left undisturbed, especially if fewer than eight healthy plants are found together.*

Magical Uses: Witches once used the root in love potions—the fresh root to encourage true love, and the withered root to abort misguided passions. These plants are said to be the food of satyrs. In Greek tradition, Orchis, the son of a nymph and a satyr, was killed for insulting a Bacchanalian priestess. His father then turned him into the flower, orchid, which bears his name.

    Burn the powdered root with musk oil for sexual passion.

Rose, *Rosa* spp.

Parts Used and Herbal Uses: Please see page 51 in "The Herbs of Meán Earraigh."

Magical Uses: The rose is an herb of love.

ROWAN, *SORBUS AUCUPARIA*

Part Used: Fruit.

Herbal Uses: Rowan is a close relative of *Sorbus americana* (American mountain ash) and can be used in the same way herbally. The bark is decocted for diarrhea and for vaginal douches; simmer two teaspoons of the bark per cup of water for twenty minutes. The bark is tinctured in alcohol for eight days to treat fevers (especially intermittent fever); follow the standard instructions for alcohol tinctures on page 15. The berries are gathered when ripe and then dried or made into jam. The berries are very high in vitamin C and are useful for sore throats and tonsillitis. Take one teaspoon of the fresh berry juice or a quarter cup of the tea made by simmering one teaspoon per cup of water for twenty minutes. The ancient Welsh made an ale from rowan berries.

Homeopathic Uses: Homeopaths use *Pyrus* (mountain ash) for eye irritation, sensations of constriction around the waist, and "cold water in the stomach" (which is coldness extending up to the esophagus), neuralgia, gout, and spasms of pain in the uterus, bladder, and heart.

Magical Uses: Rowan is primarily an herb of protection and healing. Wear a tiny cross of rowan wood somewhere in your clothing. The branches make magic wands. The leaf and berry are used in incense to increase psychic powers.

SORREL (SHAMROCK, WOOD SORREL), *OXALIS ACETOSELLA*

Parts Used: Leaf, stem, and flower.

Herbal Uses: Sorrel has sensitive leaves that fold up at night and at the threat of bad weather. Its beautiful white flowers, veined with red, bloom from May to July. Cold sorrel tea can help with heartburn and liver disorders. Steep two teaspoons per cup of water for twenty minutes; the dose is a quarter cup four times a day. Or make a tincture following the standard instructions for tinctures on page 15. Take ten to thirty drops four times a day. The leaves are eaten in soups and salads.

   CAUTION: *People with weak kidneys should avoid sorrel because of its high oxalic acid content.*

Homeopathic Uses: Homeopaths use *Oxalis acetosella* juice on cancerous growths of the lip. The fresh juice is also helpful on insect bites, stings, warts, and infected wounds.

Magical Uses: Fresh shamrocks are placed in the sickroom to bring health and healing. The dried leaf is said to bring luck, protect the heart from diseases, and enable one to see fairies.

Shamrocks are sacred to the triple Goddess. A four-leafed shamrock brings fame, wealth, faithful love, and perfect health. A five-leafed shamrock is unlucky. A two-leafed one enables the wearer to see her future lover.

WOODRUFF, *GALIUM ODORATUM, ASPERULA ODORATA*

Part Used: Leaf.

Herbal Uses: The fresh leaf is used in poultices for wounds and skin irritations; follow the standard instructions for poultices on page 15. The tea of the fresh herb is soothing to the stomach, cleans the liver, and is said to purge gravel and stones from the bladder. The fresh or dried herb has been used to treat migraine headaches and to calm hysteria and insomnia. Steep two teaspoons per cup of water for twenty minutes; take up to one cup a day in quarter-cup doses. Steep the herb in white wine to lift the spirits; this is the classic herb for May wine. The dried herb is placed in drawers and closets to repel moths.

CAUTION: *Overdose symptoms include nausea, vomiting, and dizziness.*

Magical Uses: Woodruff attracts wealth and brings victory to athletes. In ancient times, rose petals, lavender, box, and woodruff were strewn on floors and made into decorations on holy days.

CHAPTER 8

Meán Samhraidh
Summer Solstice, Midsummer

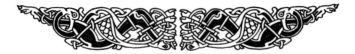

The son of the King of the Moy in Midsummer
Found a girl in the greenwood;
She gave him black fruit from thornbushes.
She gave him an armful of strawberries on rushes . . .

from Dillon, **Early Irish Literature**

At Midsummer the sun is at its zenith and we enjoy the longest day of the year. For the ancient Celts the sun was central to the activities of the ritual year. Votive models of solar worship practices have been discovered: carriages drawn by stags, oxen, or swans and filled with birds and horned animals. Sometimes the image of a God or Goddess was placed in the carriage as well.

Swans are shown pulling or perching on a carriage, often bound together with chains. The lead bird is sometimes attached to a solar symbol. Long-legged waterbirds such as cranes were associated with solar deities in the role of healing, while swans were the embodiment of purity, sensuality, love, kindliness of feeling, and magic spells cast through beautiful music. Even the raven appears as a solar bird of wisdom and prophecy.

Bulls are often connected with the swans, stags, and horses in the iconography of solar worship and seem to be associated with solar cults. The horse is sometimes shown pulling a wheeled chariot containing a solar disc, and in ancient Irish literature a great hero, heroine, or extra-ordinary horse would be compared to the sun.

The therapeutic value of the sun was associated with the healing properties of water. Solar shrines were often set up at healing springs. Water was the mystical entranceway to the Otherworld, and offerings would be thrown into wells and lakes as gifts for the Gods and God-desses. Glass, pottery, coins, stones, carved wooden figures, and golden objects found their way into the depths. Sacred wells were used for scrying, healing, and divination. On certain days wells were honored by "well dressing": the well would be covered with flowers and tree branches, circumambulated sunwise, and serenaded with music and dancing. A feast would follow, as thanksgiving for the water and the Earth Mother who provides for all. The well dressing ritual might have included a rainmaking ceremony, in which the well was petitioned three times for rain; celebrants would fill bowls of water to scatter on fields and gardens.

At midnight on the solstice, fires were lit on every hill. People danced around the fires and leapt through them. Blazing herbs from the sacred bonfire were carried to the stables to bless the cows and calves. Blazing torches were carried sunwise around the house and field. Coals from the Midsummer fire were scattered on fields to ensure a good harvest.

A "white horse" made of a long wooden frame with a horse's head and a white sheet covering was seen to "leap" through the flames to represent the beasts of the farmyard.

Tree worship played a vital role in the Midsummer festivities. Oaks near wells and fountains were decorated with colored cloths. Hawthorn trees were decked with flowers and ribbons as people danced around them. Feasting and games followed the dancing.

Bile, the progenitor and Otherworldly patriarch of the Celtic peoples, is honored at Meán Samhraidh. His consort is Danu (Anu, Ana, Don), to whom prayers for abundance and prosperity are directed on Mid-summer's Eve. Her suppliants carry torches of straw fixed on long branches to the hilltops, to bless the cattle and the newly planted corn.

Danu is linked with the rivers Danube, Dnieper, Dniester, and Don in Russia. She is the goddess of pregnancy, ripening, and the home. Mother of the Irish Gods and Goddesses and of the Tuatha Dé Danann ("the tribe of the Goddess Danu"), she is the Celtic Magna Mater who mothers the land.

So revered was she in former times that the constellation we call

"Cassiopeia's Chair" was known to the ancients as "Don's Court." The "Northern Crown" was called "Caer Arianrhod," the castle of Don's daughter. The "Milky Way" was "Castle Gwydion," the castle of Don's son. Nuada Argetlam ("of the silver hand") was lord of twenty-one thousand cattle and a God of battle and generosity. Danu was his mother.

Thus the hilltop fires and the fires of the far distant stars mirror the warmth and life-giving energies of the Great Mother, Danu.

The Herbs of Meán Samhraidh

Chamomile, Chickweed, Chicory, Cinquefoil,
Delphinium (Larkspur), Dogwood, Elderflower, Fennel,
Figwort, Hemp, Lavender, Male Fern, Meadowsweet, Mistletoe,
Mugwort, Pine, Rose, St. John's Wort, Vervain

Strew vervain or sage and tobacco on your garden as an offering to the fairies and elementals who help it grow.

Please refer to chapter 2, "Herbal Basics," for methods of preparation.

CHAMOMILE, *ANTHEMIS NOBILIS, MATRICARIA CHAMOMILLA*

Parts Used and Herbal Uses: Please see page 34 in "The Herbs of Meán Geimhridh."

Magical Uses: Chamomile, an herb of the sun, brings power and light to spells and protects the home from all dark influences.

CHICKWEED (STARWORT), *STELLARIA MEDIA*

Parts Used: Leaf and stem.

Herbal Uses: Fresh or dried chickweed is used in poultices and salves and can be eaten as a vegetable. Follow the standard instructions for salves and poultices on pages 14 and 15. A strong chickweed tea will ease constipation; take cupful doses every few hours until relief is obtained. Chickweed oil is helpful for stopping the itch of eczema. Chop the plant and grind it, cover it (just barely) with good quality olive oil, and let it sit for a few days. Strain and use. This will be most helpful for dry, itchy conditions. For "moist" eczema, use a strong wash of the tea.

Homeopathic Uses: Homeopaths use *Stellaria media* in low potencies for conditions of low metabolism, rheumatism, psoriasis, enlarged and painful liver, and constipation or alternating constipation and diarrhea. All symptoms are worse in the mornings and are aggravated by warmth and tobacco.

Magical Uses: Chickweed is an herb of love and is worn or imbibed to attract or improve a relationship.

CHICORY, *CICHORIUM INTYBUS*

Parts Used: Root and flowering herb.

Herbal Uses: The young and tender spring roots are boiled and eaten with butter, or dried, ground, and roasted to make a coffee-like brew, sometimes blended into a coffee-bean mixture. The leaves are eaten in salads—use very young plants, or blanch them by keeping the growing plants covered with a basket. The blanched herb is used like spinach or kale. Chicory can be grown during the winter in a cellar and the tender shoots eaten. Poke root (*Phylotacca americana*) can be used the same way. A decoction of chicory root helps jaundice, enlarged liver, gout, and rheumatism. Use one teaspoon per cup of water and simmer for five minutes. Strain and take up to a cup and a half per day in small doses. Steep two teaspoons per cup for twenty minutes. Take one-quarter cup, four times a day. The infused herb is used for skin eruptions associated with gout. The leaves make a poultice to soothe the eyes and inflammations in general. Follow the general instructions for poultices on page 15.

Chicory is similar to dandelion in its medicinal virtues.

CAUTION: *Overdose can cause venous congestion in the digestive tract and increased blood flow to the head. Loss of visual power in the retina can also result.*

Magical Uses: Chicory is an herb of the sun, used to transcend any obstacle that life may bring. It helps a person cultivate frugality and wins the favors of important people.

CINQUEFOIL, *POTENTILLA REPTANS, POTENTILLA CANADENSIS*

Parts Used and Herbal Uses: Please see page 48 in "The Herbs of Meán Earraigh."

Magical Uses: Cinquefoil is an herb of purification, protection, and abundance.

DELPHINIUM (LARKSPUR), *DELPHINIUM* SPP.

Part Used: Flowering herb.

Herbal Uses: The fresh juice of the leaf of *Delphinium consolida* is applied as a poultice for bleeding hemorrhoids. The infusion of the whole plant is used in colic: gather the flowering herb *before* seed formation. Steep one teaspoon of the dried herb in one cup of water for five minutes. Take one cup a day. Use the herb dried, and steep for five minutes only. Do not exceed one cup a day.

A tincture of the *Delphinium staphysagria* (stavesacre) seed is used to destroy head lice. Add a few drops to shampoo (see standard method for tincture on page 15). This herb is perhaps too powerful for internal use.

CAUTION: Delphinium consolida, *the field larkspur, is a poisonous plant, which when used wisely has curative value. The seeds if eaten cause severe vomiting and purging.*

Homeopathic Uses: Homeopaths use stavesacre for illnesses brought on by indignation. It is classic for bladder infections, prostatic problems, and pain following abdominal surgery. All symptoms are worsened by anger, mortification, and grief.

Magical Uses: Gaze at the Midsummer fires through a bunch of larkspur to strengthen the eyes. Delphinium provides generous, altruistic leadership.

DOGWOOD, *CORNUS FLORIDA*

Parts Used and Herbal Uses: Please see page 49 in "The Herbs of Meán Earraigh."

Magical Uses: Every part of the dogwood can be used as a protective charm.

ELDERFLOWER, *SAMBUCUS NIGRA*

Parts Used: Leaf, flower, and berry.

Herbal Uses: The black elder can be used as an insecticide in the garden or to repel insects from the face and body. A simple infusion of the fresh leaf is made for this purpose. It can also be poured down mouse and mole holes. The berries are used for jam, wine, pies, and syrups. Medicinally, they help coughs, colic, diarrhea, sore throats, asthma, and flu. A pinch of cinnamon makes the tea more warming. The leaves are added to salves for skin conditions. Follow the standard instructions for salves on page 14. The flowers are infused for fevers, eruptive skin conditions such as measles, and severe bronchial and lung problems. A classic flu remedy is a mixture of elderflower, yarrow, and peppermint teas. Keep the patient well covered, as the flowers promote sweating. Use two teaspoons of the herbs per cup of water, steep for twenty minutes, and take up to three cups a day.

Homeopathic Uses: Homeopaths use *Sambucus nigra* for conditions accompanied by profuse perspiration and suffocative coughs that are worse around midnight.

Magical Uses: Panpipes are made of elder stems. A dryad "Elder Mother" is said to live in the tree; she will haunt anyone who cuts down her wood. Stand or sleep under an elder on Midsummer Eve to see the King of the Fairies and his retinue pass by. The flowers are used in wish-fulfillment spells. The leaves, flowers, and berries are strewn on a person, place, or thing to bless it.

FENNEL, *FOENICULUM VULGARE*

Parts Used: Seed, root, and leaf.

Herbal Uses: To help with indigestion and gas, pour boiling water over crushed fennel seeds (one teaspoon seed to a pint of water). The seeds are simmered in syrups for coughs, shortness of breath, and wheezing. Powdered fennel seed repels fleas from pets' sleeping quarters. Place fennel inside a fish when you cook it to make it more digestible. The leaves and seeds when boiled with barley increase breast milk. The seeds and root help clean the liver, spleen, gallbladder, and blood. The tea and broth of this herb are said to help in weight loss programs. Fennel is eaten in salads, soups, and breads.

Fennel oil mixed with honey can be taken for coughs, and the tea is used as a gargle. The oil is eaten with honey to allay gas and it is applied externally to rheumatic swellings. The seeds are boiled to make an eye wash: use one-half teaspoon of seed per cup of water, three times a day, and be sure to strain carefully before use.

Magical Uses: Fennel and St. John's wort are hung over the door at Midsummer to repel evil spirits. Carry fennel to influence others to trust your words. It is used in spells for healing and purification.

FIGWORT, *SCROPHULARIA NODOSA*

Parts Used and Herbal Uses: Please see page 92 in "Herbs of the Druids."

Magical Uses: This plant is smoked in the Midsummer fire and hung in the home as an herb of health and protection.

HEMP, *CANNABIS SATIVA*

Parts Used: Seed and leaf.

Herbal Uses: Known as marijuana. The seeds have none of the intoxicating effects of the leaves and flowers. The seeds are used as a laxative for people in a weakened state (for instance, the elderly, postpartum women, the anemic, and those with high fevers). One ounce of the ground seed is simmered in one quart of water until the liquid is reduced to a pint; three doses (one-third pint each) a day are given. The leaf is used to allay the nausea associated with chemotherapy, as a tranquilizer, and for glaucoma. Smoke it or make a tea of two teaspoons per cup of water, steeped for twenty minutes. Take one-fourth cup four times a day. Painful urinary conditions, gonorrhea, and painful menstruation have been treated by it. One to three drops of the tincture of the herb, taken every three hours, has been claimed to cure gonorrhea.

  CAUTION: *This herb should be used only with medical supervision.*

Homeopathic Uses: Homeopaths use *Cannabis sativa* for stuttering, confusion of thought and speech, cataracts, burning urine, bad dreams, and oppressed breathing that is better when standing up.

Magical Uses: Hemp is added to incense, often in combination with

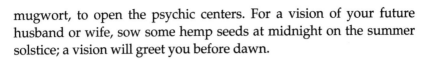

mugwort, to open the psychic centers. For a vision of your future husband or wife, sow some hemp seeds at midnight on the summer solstice; a vision will greet you before dawn.

LAVENDER, *LAVANDULA VERA*, *L. OFFICINALIS*

Parts Used: Leaf and flower.

Herbal Uses: The oil is used for intestinal gas, migraine, and dizziness. Being antiseptic, lavender is added to healing salves. Follow the standard directions for salves on page 14. A tea of the leaf allays nausea and vomiting. Use two teaspoons per cup of water and steep for twenty minutes. The dose is one-fourth cup four times a day. Steep lavender blossoms in white wine (add rose petals, if you like) for two weeks and strain to make a natural antidepressant beverage. Lavender and rose petal vinegar is applied to the temples and brow to ease headache. Lavender oil is added to footbaths, eases toothaches and sprains, and is used as a rub for hysteria and palsy.

Magical Uses: Lavender is strewn into bonfires at Midsummer as an offering to the Gods and Goddesses. An ingredient of love spells, its scent is said to attract men. Lavender in the home brings peace, joy, and healing.

MALE FERN, *DRYOPTERIS FILIX-MAS*, *ASPIDIUM FILIX-MAS*

Part Used: Root.

Herbal Uses: The fall-gathered root is a remedy for tapeworm. A few hours after it has been ingested, a purgative is given. Begin the vermifuge process by eating fresh garlic. Take one to four teaspoons of the liquid extract of the root, or of the powdered root, on an empty stomach and follow several hours later with castor oil. CAUTION: *Do not ingest alcohol while taking this herb. Overdose can result in blindness and death.*

The roots are added to healing salves for wounds and rubbed into the limbs of children with rickets. Follow the standard directions for salves on page 14.

Homeopathic Uses: Homeopaths use *Aspidium filix-mas* for tapeworm with constipation, blindness, and inflammations of the lymphatic glands.

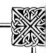

Magical Uses: The male fern brings luck and attracts women. Burn it outdoors to bring rain. The fiddleheads are dried over the Midsummer fire and used as protective amulets.

MEADOWSWEET, *Spiraea ulmaris*

Parts Used and Herbal Uses: Please see page 98 in "Herbs of the Druids."

Magical Uses: Meadowsweet is used in bridal bouquets and in love spells.

MISTLETOE, *Viscum album*

Parts Used and Herbal Uses: Please see page 100 in "Herbs of the Druids."

Magical Uses: One of the most sacred of Druid herbs, this plant helps the aspirant to perceive the Otherworld.

MUGWORT, *Artemisia vulgaris*

Parts Used: Leaf and stem.

Herbal Uses: The classic herb for premenstrual symptoms, used in tea and the bath. Use a standard infusion of two teaspoons per cup of water steeped for twenty minutes, take one-fourth cup four times a day. It makes a good foot bath for tired feet and legs. Cleansing to the liver, it promotes digestion. Mugwort is an emmenagogue, especially when combined with pennyroyal, blue cohosh, or angelica root. It is helpful in epilepsy, palsy, and hysteria and is useful for fevers. When laid among clothing, mugwort repels moths.

Homeopathic Uses: Homeopaths use *Artemisia vulgaris* for petit mal epilepsy, somnambulism, profuse perspiration that smells like garlic, and dizziness caused by colored lights. It is especially effective when given with wine.

Magical Uses: Mugwort is said to protect travelers from fatigue, sunstroke, wild animals, and evil spirits. A crown of it is worn at Midsummer. A tea or a pillow of it brings vivid prophetic dreams and helps one to contact the astral realm. Use the tea and incense to help in scrying. Use it to wash magic mirrors and crystal balls.

PINE, *PINUS* SPP.

Parts Used and Herbal Uses: Please see page 37 in "The Herbs of Meán Geimhridh."

Magical Uses: Pine is a tree of peace and immortality.

ROSE, *ROSA* SPP.

Parts Used and Herbal Uses: Please see page 51 in "The Herbs of Meán Earraigh."

Magical Uses: Roses are an herb of love.

ST. JOHN'S WORT, *HYPERICUM PERFORATUM*

Parts Used: Leaf and stem.

Herbal Uses: The herb is the part used for lung problems, bladder complaints, diarrhea, dysentery, depression, hemorrhages, and jaundice. Steep two teaspoons of the herb per cup of water for twenty minutes. Take one-half cup in the morning and one-half cup at bed time. Bed-wetting is helped by a nightly cup of the tea. The oil and fomentation are applied externally to injuries, especially when nerve endings are involved (i.e., fingers and toes), and to soften tumors and caked breasts.

To make the oil, cover the flowers with good, cold-pressed olive oil and leave the sealed preparation in the hot sun for twenty-one days or until it becomes a rich red. The oil is excellent for massages, as it affects the spine directly. Varicose veins, mild burns, inflammations, neuralgia, and rheumatism are helped by a poultice of it.

CAUTION: *Malignant tumors must be treated with care. Never rub or massage a malignant growth, as cells may become detached and travel to other parts of the body.*

Homeopathic Uses: Homeopaths use *Hypericum* for puncture wounds, surgery, nerve injury, asthma that is worsened by changes of weather or before storms, tetanus, neuritis, and chronic drowsiness. The symptoms are relieved by bending the head backwards and worsened by cold, damp, and touch.

Magical Uses: The Welsh called this plant the "leaf of the blessed." It was understood to be an ideal combination of water and fire, the ultimate healing essence. Fire symbolized the fruitful light-filled forces of summer, and water the gathering and settling forces of the dark season. Midsummer was the time of balance between these forces of light and dark.

In Brittany the plant is still ritually gathered by people wearing loose, flowing clothing. One must pray and ask permission before plucking it with the left hand. The earth around the plant is first loosened with a knife, and the whole plant is pulled out at once. Great care is taken to ensure that the roots are intact and undisturbed. The picking of this herb symbolizes the dismemberment of the God, the Summer Lord. It is a solemn sacrifice.

After drying or tincturing the plant is administered to the sick. When you give this plant to one who is sick, you are re-membering the God: putting back together the pieces of his body that have been scattered.

The mere scent of this plant causes evil spirits to fly away. It is picked at Midsummer and dried over the Midsummer fire. Use it to keep madness at bay and to keep all evil forces from the home.

VERVAIN, *VERBENA OFFICINALIS*

Parts Used and Herbal Uses: Please see page 109 in "Herbs of the Druids."

Magical Uses: Vervain is traditionally gathered at Midsummer or at the rising of the Dog Star when neither sun nor moon are in the sky. It is a sacred herb of purification.

CHAPTER 9

Lugnasad

Lammas

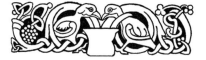

Each smooth nut puts forth its shell at the end of its branch on the margin of the corn land: the yellow grain dons its husk underneath a fresh bending brake.

from Dillon, **Early Irish Literature**

Lugnasad marks the beginning of the sun's descent into the dark of winter. It was first celebrated at Tailltean, the burial place of Lugh's foster-mother, Tailtiu. The festival is typically celebrated with races and circular dances that are designed to strengthen the community, the sun, and the land by sympathetic magic.

This is the season when the sun consummates its union with the earth, producing the first fruits of the harvest. It is an especially auspicious time for weddings.

Lugnasad is essentially a time of tension, when the dark days of winter are looming and the harvest is not quite safely in. The God of the harvest is known as the Green Man or John Barleycorn. He sacrifices himself each year so that the great cycle of life in the human community can continue. The honoring of the first fruits of the harvest eases anxiety over the fate of the crop and brings about gratitude for the impending harvest.

Lugnasad is traditionally a communal gathering held near a distinctive natural feature such as a sacred tree, an ancient cairn, a holy well, or a hilltop. Pagan deities such as Dánu and Lugh are invoked and petitioned for the protection and safety of the near-ripened crops.

At this festival, the first grain is ceremonially cut at dawn and placed on a rock in the sun to dry. Later, it is husked by hand, winnowed, ground in a quern (hand mill), kneaded on a sheepskin, and baked into bannock, which is toasted on a fire of rowan branches (or any other of the sacred woods). The bannock is broken and distributed to the assembly as the celebrants walk *deosil* (sunwise) around the fire.

On the first day of the wheat harvest the family dresses in formal attire to salute the Harvest God. Taking off his or her hat, the head of the clan faces the sun and cuts a handful of grain, whirls it three times sunwise overhead, and praises the Harvest God as the entire family joins in. Thanks are given for grain and bread, meat and wool, health, peace, and prosperity.

In some places, Lugnasad is marked by the climbing of mountains, the visiting of holy wells, and horse racing. A traditional Welsh harvest game, *rhibo*, is played by three pairs who stand facing each other, holding hands. A person is laid on their outstretched arms and tossed repeatedly in the air.*

When the harvest is done, the last sheaf is ritually cut down by all the reapers, who stand at a distance and take turns throwing sickles at it until its "neck" is finally cut. The grain is sometimes tied to look like an animal. The reaper who succeeds in "decapitating" the sheaf is honored at the harvest feast.

The last sheaf is sometimes fashioned into a "corn dolly" dressed as a young woman if the harvest is good or a *cailleach* (hag or death crone) if the harvest is poor. The dolly is displayed at the harvest supper.

The last load of grain is sometimes accompanied by a "Harvest Lord" and "Harvest Queen," who sit on it as it is carted home in a wagon decorated with flowers and branches. The last sheaf is waved aloft while spectators attempt to drench the cart with water. It is considered very good luck to get the wagon home dry.

The reaper who carries the sheaf into the farmhouse is met by a woman carrying a bucket of water. She attempts to pour the water on him, and his reward for staying dry is a kiss. If he gets wet, the bucket is placed over his head.

---

* This game emulates the act of winnowing grain by tossing it so that the chaff can be blown away.

The last sheaf might stand in the kitchen or on the mantle until the next harvest. It might be placed in the fork of a tree or mixed with the seed for the next year's sowing. Sometimes it is plowed back into the soil, or left in a field to rot away. It can be ritually burned after the next year's harvest, or given to a prized animal as fodder. In this way, the fertilizing spirit of the Harvest God is passed from harvest to harvest.

A medieval poem describes the fate of those who neglect the Lugnasad assembly:

> There comes for neglect of it
> Baldness, weakness, early greyness
> Kings without keenness or jollity
> Without hospitality or truth.

from Rees and Rees, **Celtic Heritage**

By observing the Lugnasad assembly, the people are assured of plentiful wheat and milk, protection from conquest, just laws, comfort in the home, and a good harvest of fruit and fish.

The traditional festival is a time for horse races, chariot races, musical contests, poetry competitions, bestowal of new ranks and honors, and weddings. Violence, enmity between wives and husbands, and the levying of debts are forbidden.

Dánu, the Earth Mother, is of course honored at the rites. The male aspect of deity who is honored at Lugnasad is Lugh Samildánach, master of arts and patron of scholars, craftsmen, warriors, and magicians. Lugh is known as an "all-purpose" God of extraordinary intellectual ability. He is a powerful magician whose spells can affect the outcome of battles.

He is usually pictured with a mighty spear or as a youth accompanied by ravens, symbols of wisdom and prophecy. An old story relates how Lugh was the surviving brother of three born simultaneously, hinting at his possible origins as a triple-god figure.

When Lugh attempted to enter the great hall of the Tuatha Dé Danaan, he was turned away by the gatekeeper because they already had a smith, a great war hero, a harper, a poet, a historian, a doctor, and a magus. Lugh then asked if they had any individual in the tribe who could do *all* those things. When they said no, Lugh announced that he was master of every one of those arts, and so he was granted admittance.

THE HERBS OF LUGNASAD

Berries, Fenugreek, Frankincense, Heather,
Hollyhock, Mistletoe, Oak, Oat, Sunflower

Bake some berry pies in honor of the harvest and share them with your friends. Vegetables of all kinds are placed on the altar and used as decorations at Lugnasad. Of course, you will offer up only the very best specimens from the garden.

Please refer to chapter 2, "Herbal Basics," for methods of preparation.

BERRIES

Magical Uses: Pies made of berries are baked to commemorate the death of the God, the "Green Man," who lives in all vegetation and who is sacrificed each year at the harvest so that the greater life may prosper.

FENUGREEK, *Trigonella foenum-graecum*

Part Used: Seed.

Herbal Uses: The seeds are nutritious and tonic. The powdered seed is taken for osteomyelitis, scrofula, and tuberculosis. It prevents fever, strengthens the stomach and digestion, and helps diabetics regulate insulin. Anemia and weakness of all kinds can be addressed by this herb. The dose is three to nine grams. The powdered seed is used in poultices for boils, abscesses, tumors, swollen glands, and sores. Follow the standard directions for poultices given on page 15. Use the tea for bronchitis, sore throats, and fevers. Steep two teaspoons in one cup of cold water for five hours, then boil for one minute. Take up to three cups a day. Peppermint or lemon will improve the taste. Fenugreek is reputed to be an aphrodisiac.

Magical Uses: Fenugreek used in rinse water as you clean, or placed around the house, will attract money. Place some in a jar and add a bit to your cache daily. When your objective is achieved, bury the seeds in the earth. The herb is sacred to Apollo.

Frankincense (Olibanum), *Boswellia thuriferia,* *Boswellia carterii*

Part Used and Herbal Uses: Please see page 35 in "The Herbs of Meán Geimhridh."

Magical Uses: Frankincense is an herb of purification, protection, and exorcism. Its use is said to accelerate spiritual growth and to eliminate unwanted influences.

Heather, *Calluna vulgaris*

Parts Used and Herbal Uses: Please see page 43 in "The Herbs of Imbolc/Oimealg."

Magical Uses: Heather is an herb of luck and protection used in rainmaking ceremonies.

Hollyhock, *Althaea rosea*

Part Used: Flower.

Herbal Uses: Hollyhock flowers are gathered in July and August when they are in full bloom. Their actions are cooling and soothing to the mucous membranes. Mouth and throat irritations and inflammations of the neck of the bladder are helped. Steep two teaspoons of the flowers per cup of water for twenty minutes. Take one-fourth cup four times a day.

Homeopathic Uses: Homeopaths use a relative of hollyhock, *Althaea officinalis* (marshmallow) for irritable bladder, throat, and bronchi.

Magical Uses: Hollyhock flowers attract money, success, and material wealth of all kinds. They are favored by the fairies who bring luck to the home. Plant some by *your* home!

Mistletoe, *Viscum album*

Parts Used and Herbal Uses: Please see page 100 in "Herbs of the Druids."

Magical Uses: This herb is used to strengthen all magical workings and especially for healing, protection, and beautiful dreams.

OAK, *QUERCUS* SPP.

Parts Used and Herbal Uses: See page 23 in "The Herbs of Samhain."

Magical Uses: The oak is a tree of strength, perseverance, and protection. It brings fertility to ideas, projects, and harvest magic.

OAT, *AVENA SATIVA*

Parts Used: Grain and straw.

Herbal Uses: The tincture forms the basis of all nerve tonics. Oatmeal, easily digested, is ideal food for invalids, postpartum women, and those with fevers. Add dates or raisins to the oats as they cook for extra nutrition. Cooked oats thickened with slippery elm powder (*Ulmus fulva*) make a poultice for skin irritations. The tincture strengthens the uterus. Follow the standard directions for tincture on page 15. A tea of oat straw helps chest complaints. Simmer small pieces of the straw in water for one hour, and add honey. A bath of it benefits rheumatism, lumbago, paralysis, liver and kidney disease, bladder problems, colic, bedwetting, chronically tired and cold feet, skin diseases, frostbite, wounds, and eye problems. Boil about two pounds of the straw in three quarts of water for thirty minutes and add to the bath. Eating oats lowers cholesterol.

Homeopathic Uses: Homeopaths use *Avena sativa* for colds with acute mucus discharge, exhaustion, nerve tremors, paralysis, epilepsy, sleeplessness, and the bad effects of morphine.

Magical Uses: Oat cakes are made with the new grain and shared with family and friends at Lugnasad. In olden times, they were ground in a quern and baked on a sheepskin next to the fire. Oats are used in money spells.

SUNFLOWER, *HELIANTHUS ANNUS*

Part Used: Seed.

Herbal Uses: Sunflower, a New World plant, has only recently entered the neo-Pagan tradition. Sunflower seeds are simmered in water (one ounce seed to one quart of liquid) until half of the water is absorbed or evaporated. Add six ounces of gin as a preservative, and honey to taste. The preparation is a good syrup for lung and throat problems, coughs, and colds. The oil can be used for the same conditions: ten to fifteen drops, three times per day. A tea of the toasted seed has been used for whooping cough. A tincture of the seed has been used to treat fevers, and it is a substitute for quinine. The leaves are smoked in herbal tobacco mixtures.

Homeopathic Uses: Homeopaths use the remedy *Helianthus* for spleen afflictions, intermittent fever, catarrhal conditions, nasal hemorrhages, nausea, and vomiting. Black stool, dry mouth, red hot skin, and vomiting are guiding symptoms. Helianthus is used externally as a wound remedy in the same ways that one would use arnica or calendula tinctures and salves.

Magical Uses: In the Aztec temples of the sun, priestesses carried sunflowers and wore them as crowns. As sun symbols, these flowers symbolize the healthy ego, the wisdom, and the fertility of the solar logos.

CHAPTER 10

Meán Fómhair
Fall Equinox

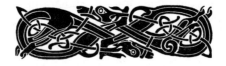

A tree of apples—great its bounty!
Like a hostel, vast!
A pretty bush, thick as a fist, of tiny hazelnuts
A green mass of branches.

from Dillon, **Early Irish Literature**

The autumn equinox is a special moment when night and day are of equal length, and we pause to pay respects to the impending dark. Equally so, we pause to thank the waning sunlight for its life-nourishing gifts—the harvest that we see around us and the abundance and wealth of our family and clan.

An ancient symbol for the wealth of the harvest is the cornucopia—the horn of plenty—which is both male (phallic) and female (hollow and receptive). Hermaphroditic images were familiar to the ancient Europeans; images such as the one found at the Bell Trackway in Somerset, England, were figures with both breasts and a phallus. Horned Goddesses have been discovered in European excavations.*

At Meán Fómhair we honor also the God of the forest, the Green Man, by offering libations to trees. Such gifts as cider, wine, herbs, and fertilizer are appropriate at this time. Offerings are scattered, in a spirit of thanksgiving, over the harvested fields.

The essential nature of this feast is the drawing together and drawing

---

* For an excellent discussion of these, see Marija Gimbutas, *The Gods and Goddesses of Old Europe, 7000-3500 B.C.*

in of the family as it prepares to face the chaos of the season of Samhain. Meán Fómhair provides a last chance to finish the old business of summer so that the dark season can be passed as a time of reflection and peace. At this festival, it is appropriate to wear lavish finery and rich fabrics in sumptuous settings. The best tableware and the finest foods are displayed as mead and music fill the house with cheer.

We bid farewell to the strength of Lugh and welcome once again the power of the Cailleach, the Old One, the hag and crone. She is the Dark Woman who visits us with gifts of wisdom and insight. She is the triple Goddess who appears at the deaths of kings, queens, and heroes. She is the Great Queen who gives birth and reaps death; the mystical embodiment of the land.

THE HERBS OF MEÁN FÓMHAIR

Acorn, Benzoin, Fern, Grains, Honeysuckle (Woodbine),
Marigold, Milkweed, Myrrh, Passionflower, Rose,
Sage, Solomon's Seal, Thistle, Vegetables

Grains of all kinds are baked into breads and cakes and shared at fall equinox gatherings. Baked goods made with new grain are eaten in honor of the Green Man, the living spirit of the vegetation, who sacrifices himself in autumn so that other lives may carry on. Though he may appear to die at Samhain, by Yule he is reconceived as light, to appear again in material form in the spring. Bake some bread of the new grain harvest and share it with your friends. The very best produce from field and forest is placed on the altar at Meán Fómhair. We give thanks to the fairies and the elementals who helped the garden grow. It is considered wise to pick one of each flower and vegetable of the harvest (choose only the very best specimens, free of blemish or blight) and leave it on an outdoor shrine for the nature spirits in thanks for their kind work all summer.

Please refer to chapter 2, "Herbal Basics," for methods of preparation.

ACORN, QUERCUS SPP.

Parts Used and Herbal Uses: Please see page 23 in "The Herbs of Samhain."

Magical Uses: Acorns bring fertility to every sphere of life. Wear them, carry them, and use them to decorate the altar.

BENZOIN, *STYRAX BENZOIN*

Part Used: Resin.

Herbal Uses: A tree resin used externally, diluted with water, as an antiseptic skin wash. Taken internally, it relieves intestinal gas and is antiseptic to the urinary tract. Take ten to twenty drops in water or tea four times a day. Put it in vaporizers or use it as an inhalant for bronchitis and laryngitis. A simple method is to place it, along with a few drops of the oils of peppermint and eucalyptus, in a bowl of boiling hot water. Put your face as close to the bowl as you can and cover your head, and the bowl, with a towel. Inhale the steam. Tincture of benzoin is often added to salves as a preservative: (one ounce of benzoin to about one and a half quarts of salve). (See page 14 for directions for making salves.)

Homeopathic Uses: Homeopaths use *Benzoicum acidum* (benzoic acid), the active constituent of benzoin, for kidney problems with offensive urine, offensive liquid stool, and pain in the Achilles tendon. All symptoms are worse in the open air and when the body is uncovered.

Magical Uses: An herb of purification, burned in incense to sanctify an area. The scent is also used to attract business when combined with basil, peony, or cinnamon.

FERN

Parts Used: Leaf and root.

Herbal Uses: Please see Male Fern, page 71 in "The Herbs of Meán Samhraidh." Numerous ferns are used in herbal medicines. *Aspidium spinulosum*, the shield fern, is used similarly to the male fern. The leaf of *Asplenium ceterach*, spleenwort, is used in infusion to cure enlarged spleen. The leaf of *Asplenium adiantum nigrum*, black spleenwort, is used in decoction for coughs and as a hair rinse. The leaf of *Asplenium rutamuraria*, wall rue, is taken as tea for coughs, jaundice, spleen problems, kidney stones, and shortness of breath. The leaf of *Asplenium trichomanes*, common maidenhair, is used for lung ailments and as a laxative. Fronds of *Adiantum capillus-veneris*, true maidenhair, are also used for lung conditions in tea or syrup and to help the liver in jaundice. Useful in cases of kidney stones, it is said to restore fallen hair (*A. pedatum* is an American variety, with similar virtues). The fronds of *Asplenium scolopendrium* are given in infusion for diarrhea and dysentery, and in salves for burns and hemorrhoids. They also clean the liver and spleen. For the above ferns infuse one ounce of the fern leaves in one pint of water and steep for twenty minutes. Take one-fourth cup four times a day. For fern roots, simmer two teaspoons per cup for twenty minutes and take one-fourth cup four times per day. For salves follow the standard directions on page 14. *Pteris aquilina*, bracken fern, is eaten as a vegetable when the fronds are uncoiled in spring. Its roots are boiled in mead to kill intestinal worms and to benefit the spleen. The roots are used in salves, and the root powder is applied to ulcers and wounds. *Polypodium vulgare*, common poly-pody, is used in a decoction for whooping cough. The fronds are cut and dried in autumn and boiled as needed. The fresh root helps de-pression, jaundice, edema, and rheumatism. *Osmunda regalis*, royal fern, has roots that are used in salves and decocted to treat jaundice. The young fronds are used in healing ointments. *Ophioglossum vulga-tum*, adder's tongue, is taken fresh as a juice of the leaf for internal in-juries, and the leaves are also used in salves. *Botrychium lunaria*, moonwort, has fronds that are used like those of adder's tongue.

Magical Uses: Fern "seeds" are said to render one invisible if gathered on Midsummer's Eve. Ferns are also said to be an herb of immortal-ity. Moonwort is especially effective if gathered by moonlight. This fern aids in opening locks and breaking charms, is used in love spells, and has the alchemical reputation of being an herb to convert quick-silver into silver. Use it to conjure money.

HONEYSUCKLE (WOODBINE), *LONICERA CAPRIFOLIUM*

Parts Used and Herbal Uses: Please see page 50 in "The Herbs of Meán Earraigh."

Magical Uses: Honeysuckle attracts money and enhances psychic abilities.

MARIGOLD, *CALENDULA OFFICINALIS*

Parts Used and Herbal Uses: Please see page 60 in "The Herbs of Beltaine."

Magical Uses: Calendula helps one to win a court case. It encourages prophetic dreams and makes them come true.

MILKWEED, *ASCLEPIAS SYRIACA*

Parts Used: Flower bud, sap, root.

Herbal Uses: The root is said to produce temporary sterility if taken as tea. The fresh, milky juice can be dropped onto warts to make them disappear. The young green flower buds can be eaten steamed or sauteed; they taste a little like broccoli. The powder of the root and the infusion of it have been used to relieve cough and pain in cases of asthma and typhus and are also used for scrofula (tuberculosis inflammation and ulceration of the lymph nodes). Mix equal parts of the root with marshmallow root (*althea*), steep one teaspoon per cup of water, and take one-quarter cup four times a day.

    CAUTION: *This plant is poisonous if overused.*

Homeopathic Uses: Homeopaths use *Asclepias syriaca cornuti* (silkweed or milkweed) for afflictions of the nerves and the urinary tract and for pressing down uterine pains. *Asclepias tuberosa* (pleurisy root) is used for bronchitis, the pain of pleurisy, and mucus-ridden dysentery with rheumatic pain over the whole body. It has a special affinity for the chest muscles.

Magical Uses: In India, *Asclepias acida*, with its hallucinogenic juice, is considered an incarnation of Soma, a Vedic God. Soma is also the name of a sacred drink that is described in the Rig Veda. According to tradition, the Gods in heaven drink its juice, as do humans. It was the drink that influenced Indra to create Heaven and Earth. Soma is the king of plants, able to bestow health, long life, and immortality.

    Monarch butterflies and fairies are fond of milkweed. Place it in the garden to attract them.

MYRRH, *COMMIPHORA MYRRHA*

Parts Used and Herbal Uses: Please see page 44 in the "The Herbs of Imbolc/Oimealg."

Magical Uses: Myrrh enhances contemplation and meditation. Use it to bring peace, healing, and blessings to any situation.

PASSIONFLOWER, *PASSIFLORA INCARNATA*

Parts Used: Plant, flower.

Herbal Uses: The dried herb is used for insomnia, Parkinson's disease, epilepsy and other seizure disorders, hysteria, shingles, and nervous conditions of all types. The heart and liver are affected by this cooling tonic. It is also used for diarrhea and dysentery, for its calming antispasmodic and sedative effects. Passionflower may be combined with valerian, skullcap, lady's slipper, black cohosh, or hops for stress relief. Remember to avoid constipation and a diet rich in sugars, caffeine, and fats, as these further add to emotional stress.

Homeopathic Uses: Homeopaths use *Passiflora incarnata* for restlessness, exhaustion, insomnia, worry, overwork, convulsions, nocturnal coughs, and asthma.

Magical Uses: Brought into the home, passionflower calms and brings peace. Sprinkle it over the doorstep to keep harm from entering. Carry it to win friends and increase charisma. Place it in power bundles and love spells to attract love. Burn it in incense to promote understanding.

ROSE, *ROSA* SPP.

Parts Used and Herbal Uses: Please see page 61 in "The Herbs of Beltaine."

Magical Uses: Roses are an herb of love.

SAGE, *SALVIA OFFICINALIS*

Parts Used and Herbal Uses: Please see page 28 in "The Herbs of Samhain."

Magical Uses: Sage brings wisdom, immortality, and wealth.

SOLOMON'S SEAL, *POLYGONATUM OFFICINALE, P. MULTIFLORUM*

Part Used: Root.

Herbal Uses: This is an endangered species. Gather it with reverence and *only when you find a large patch* (take only a few; leave at least seven healthy plants). The part used is the root. The roots are mashed with a little cream and made into a poultice for black eyes, bruises, and sprains. Mixed with powdered slippery elm bark, they make a poultice for fresh wounds. Solomon's seal is a useful herb for lung disease, especially when there is bleeding in the lung. The dose is six to fifteen grams. It is healing and soothing to the intestinal tract and is given for hemorrhoids, chronic dysentery, tuberculosis, and heart conditions. One ounce of the root can be simmered in one pint of water for twenty minutes and given in quarter-cup doses, four times a day. The leaves are simmered into salves (see page 14 for instructions on how to make salves). The roots are mashed and simmered in wine and given to humans or animals to promote bone healing. The young roots may be eaten as a vegetable (*P. biflorum*, an American Solomon's seal, has the same medicinal and nutritional properties).

Magical Uses: Solomon's seal is sprinkled in corners to exorcise unwanted spirits. It is an herb of cleansing and consecration. Add it to incense on the altar.

THISTLES

Many thistles are used herbally, but the three given here are perhaps the best known.

BLESSED THISTLE, *CARDUUS BENEDICTUS = CNICUS BENEDICTUS = CARBENIA BENEDICTA*

Parts Used and Herbal Uses: Please see page 34 in "The Herbs of Meán Geimhridh."

Magical Uses: Thistles bestow energy and strength. Worn or placed in the home, they ward off thieves.

TEASEL, *DIPSACUS SYLVESTRIS, D. FULLONIUM*

Part Used: Root.

Herbal Uses: Teasel roots are used in salves for fistulas, cankers and warts (see page 14 for instructions in making salves). It is an herb for opening and cleansing the liver, and it helps in jaundice. Two teaspoons of the root are simmered in one cup of water, and one-fourth cup is taken four times a day. The traditional use of the dried flower heads is in fleecing wool.

Homeopathic Uses: The homeopathic tincture of *Dipsacus* is used for anal fistula and skin inflammations. It is made from the fresh plant in flower.

MILK THISTLE, *CARDUUS MARIANUS*, *SYLYBUM MARIANUM*

Parts Used: Seed, leaf, stem, and root.

Herbal Uses: Milk thistle is known as a powerful liver cleanser and re-generator and has been used to save victims of mushroom poisoning. The seeds are tinctured and the root is simmered in standard decoction to protect the liver; one-fourth cup of the decoction or five drops of the seed tincture are taken four times a day. The seeds are boiled to promote breast milk, and the poultice of the whole plant has been used externally for cancer. Milk thistle is one of the best herbs to cure depression. The young plant is eaten in spring as a blood cleanser.

CHAPTER 11

Herbs of the Druids

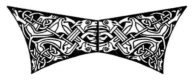

*Brooklime (Water Pimpernel), Figwort, Madder (Dyer's Weed),
Mandrake, Meadowsweet (Queen-of-the-Meadow,
Bride of the Meadow, Bridewort), Mint (Wild Mint, Marsh Mint,
Hairy Mint, Water Mint), Mistletoe (Birdlime, Golden Bough,
Holy Wood), Oak Tree (Duir), Selago, Self-Heal (All-Heal,
Heart-of-the-Earth), Vervain (Enchanter's Herb, Herb-of-Grace),
Water Horehound (Gipsyweed), Wild Basil, Woad*

Please refer to chapter 2, "Herbal Basics," for methods of preparation.

The evidence for herbs used by Druids is painfully meager. Ancient Irish law texts make references to "herb-gardens" (*lubgort*) attached to farmyards, but few herbs are mentioned. Woad (*Isatis tinctoria*) (Gaelic, *glasen*) and madder (*Rubia tinctorum*) (Gaelic, *roid*) are among them. Dr. Fergus Kelly of Institiuid Ard-Leinn Bhaile Atha Cliath (The Dublin Institute for Advanced Studies) has mentioned several herbs found in the medicolegal texts dealing with illegal injuries.* Apparently there is reference to "three foreign herbs" used for healing facial wounds: *sraif* (for

---

* Dr. Fergus Kelly is currently working on a book entitled *Early Irish Farming: The Evidence of the 7th–8th Century Law-Texts*, and he was kind enough to share this information with me in a letter.

healing the wound), *lungait* (for the color of the wound), and *argatlium* (for the skin). Lacking conclusive evidence, it has been suggested that sraif may be rue (*Ruta graveolens*). *Argatlium* could be a variation on *argatliub*, "silver-plant," which might be wormwood (*Artemisia absinthium*). No one seems to have any idea about *lungait*.*

As in all areas of particularly important knowledge, the Druids did not leave written accounts of their medicinal lore. Broadly based evidence indicates that oral traditions are handed down for centuries, remarkably intact. Writing something down, however, makes it available to anyone who sees it, regardless of their preparation and training. Once a subject is committed to paper (or parchment or stone), one has lost control over where it goes, who uses it, and in what manner.

There is also the problem of others copying the information and altering it deliberately or simply misinterpreting the data. Reading and writing can discourage thinking because the uninitiated reader might decide that the information presented—even incorrect or incomplete renderings—is final, "etched in stone."

The less charitable view is that the Druids chose to keep a monopoly on their own wisdom. Yet we know that they were avid teachers and maintained schools for men and women.

Whatever the reason for their strictly oral transmissions, the result is that most of what we have to go on is a handful of references from authors such as Pliny and Julius Caesar. It stands to reason that the Druids of Britain, Gaul, Iberia, or any other land would have used whichever local herbs were medicinally active. Hence, a good working knowledge of Western herbology is a must for any aspiring Druid of today.

The herbs presented in this chapter would have been some of the medicines of the Druids of the Northern European region.

BROOKLIME (WATER PIMPERNEL), *VERONICA BECCABUNGA*

Part Used: Above-ground portions of the herb.

A common herb of Great Britain, the Highlands, the Shetlands, Ireland, and the Channel Islands. Brooklime is found in stream beds and wet areas, along with watercress and water mint. It has a hollow, tender stem that creeps along the ground, rooting at intervals. At differ-

---

* For a discussion of rue and wormwood, please refer to "The Herbs of Samhain" in chapter 3 and to chapter 14, "Last Rites and the Celtic Otherworld."

ent points, it sends up stalks with oblong, slightly toothed leaves, which are opposite, thick, and shiny. The flowers are bright blue (occasionally pink) and occur in pairs.

This plant was ritually gathered, according to Pliny, by a Druid who first spent several days fasting and then dug up the plant by its roots with the left hand. The herb was placed in a drinking trough used by cattle (perhaps to keep it moist), after which it was used as a healing agent.

Herbal Uses: The plant is antiscorbutic (prevents scurvy) and was once eaten in salads. Brooklime and watercress are often found together, and they were both collected in spring as vegetables.* The fresh leaves can be used, mashed, as a poultice for burns, itching, and wounds. (See page 15 for directions on how to make poultices.) The juice of the fresh plant, being high in vitamin C, is used in spring tonics. It is diuretic and is taken in one- to three-tablespoon doses three times a day in a standard infusion of two teaspoons per cup, steeped for twenty minutes. Those with sensitive stomachs can take it in milk.

The infusion is used as a blood cleanser, to break up and pass kidney stones, and to treat anemia and fevers. It brings on menstruation and helps expel a dead fetus. The herb is heated with oil and vinegar and applied to tumors and swellings.

CAUTION: *Pregnant women should avoid this plant.*

Magical Uses: Brooklime is considered an herb of Mars because of its hot and biting nature. It is often combined with watercress, which is used by those wishing to keep safe in boats or while crossing bodies of water. It is eaten at dawn to improve one's visionary capacities and to strengthen the power and objectivity of the "third eye."

FIGWORT, *Scrophularia nodosa*

Parts Used: Above-ground portions of herb, and root.

A plant resembling figwort seems to have been used by the Druids. Figwort is an important medicinal, common in moist areas and damp woods of the British Isles. It has a square stem, oval to lanceolate leaves, and opposite purple flowers. It attains a height of two to four feet. The leaves and tubers have an unpleasant smell.

---

* Native Americans also used to keep track of patches of watercress, and in winter, when ice covered the streams, they would break through to get the fresh, green plants. This was a way to get fresh greens and vitamins in the deepest winter.

Herbal Uses: The root is important for diabetes, tuberculosis, long-lasting low-grade fevers and other wasting conditions, sore throats, and edema. It clears the glandular system and the liver, thus relieving skin eruptions and liver conditions. Simmer two teaspoons of the root per cup of water for twenty minutes. Take one-fourth cup per day, four times a day.

As an external poultice, the root treats ringworm, bruises, hemorrhoids, swellings, and itchy eruptions. The whole herb is used externally as a poultice to dissolve clotted blood and for tumors, wens, eczema, scabies, rashes, and the like. It has been added to salves and ointments for wounds and bruises. The leaves are used on burns and swellings. (See pages 14 and 15 for directions on how to make salves, poultices, and tinctures.) The tincture is taken twenty drops at a time and can be used both internally and externally.

Used internally or externally as a tea, poultice, or tincture, the plant is rich in manganese, making it a powerful skin healer. The tea is taken for tumors of all kinds.

The herb and root have been used to treat cancer of the fleshy parts. The powdered root in water has been used as a tea to treat condyloma. The juice of the root and leaf are applied externally to tumors and cancers. The ointment treats painful tumors, and the fresh poultice may be used for inflamed tumors and glandular indurations. When figwort is used externally, the tea is also given internally as further therapeutic support.*

Homeopathic Uses: Homeopaths use *Scrophularia nodosa* for Hodgkin's disease and conditions with enlarged glands, for breast tumors, eczema of the ear, scrofula, painful hemorrhoids, and skin cancer. All symptoms are worse when the patient lies on the right side.

Magical Uses: Figwort is an herb of Venus. It is worn as a protective herb and is placed in the home to attract health, peace, and joy.

At Midsummer, the ancient Gauls would light fires on the hilltops to bring healing and protection to the crops, animals, and people. These fires mirrored the power of Belenos, the God of the Sun. Herbs were ritually smoked in these fires and later used as amulets and

---

* Other herbs used in poultices for tumors and cancer are slippery elm (bark, leaf, and root), heather (flowers and twigs), maple leaf (powder), and speedwell (*Veronica officinalis*), which is especially well suited to breast cancers. The fresh juice of veronica benefits all internal cancers. Mandrake (leaf and root) is crushed and boiled and applied to tumors. Chaparral (powder) is especially well suited to skin cancers.

protective decorations for the house and barn. The herbs thus prepared included figwort, ivy, mugwort, yarrow, vervain, elder, fennel, chamomile, melilot, St. John's wort, plantain, hawthorn, lavender, and male fern.

MADDER (DYER'S WEED), *RUBIA TINCTORUM*

Part Used: Root.

This plant may grow to a height of eight feet; yet it produces stems so weak that it often lies on the ground. The stalks are prickly, and the leaves have spines on the midrib along the underside. The paired flowers are yellow, appear after the second or third year, and are followed by small black berries. Madder is found in the south of England and in Europe.

Herbal Uses: The part used is the root, which is gathered when the plant is three to six years old. It is especially useful in urinary tract afflictions in which the system has become alkaline. Madder stops bleeding and inflammations and cleanses the blood. It has been used to hasten the healing of broken bones, for diarrhea, and for fevers. It colors milk and urine red when ingested as a tea, and helps to bring on the menses. Steep one teaspoon of the fresh or dry root in one cup of water for twenty minutes. Take up to one and a half cups per day.

Madder has a marked effect on the liver and has been found useful in jaundice. Skin conditions benefit from the root, which is used fresh or dry in infusions. Two ounces of the root can be boiled in six quarts of water and added to the tub to make a bath that will heal the skin.

Madder is used to dye wool, cotton, linen, silk, and leather. Different mordants will bring out different shades of crimson. Alum is used to bring out a lacquer red; chrome gives the dye a garnet color; alum and tannic acid together create red. Tin produces orange, and iron, brown.

Homeopathic Uses: Homeopaths use *Rubia tinctorum* (the tincture of madder) for spleen ailments.

Magical Uses: Make a gift to a young woman of skeins of wool or a garment of natural cloth dyed with madder, for her coming-of-age ceremony. Madder is an herb of Mars.

MANDRAKE, *MANDRAGORA OFFICINALIS, M. VERNALIS, M. AUTUMNALIS*

> Not poppy, nor mandragora,
> Nor all the drowsy syrups of the world,
> Shall ever medicine thee to that sweet sleep
> Which thou ow'dst yesterday.
>
> **Othello,** *Act III, scene III*

Part Used: Root.

Ancient Greeks, Egyptians, and Arabs used this herb. A native of southern Europe, it figures prominently in the Western European magical tradition. We know that the early Greek temples of healing used henbane (*Hyoscyamus niger*) and mandrake to induce a healing sleep.

Because of the high level of commerce between ancient peoples and the evidence that Druids visited Greece in the time of Pythagoras, it is highly likely that the knowledge of this plant was widely disseminated.

One of the most fascinating uses of mandrake seems to have been its ability to engender shamanic trances. *M. officinalis, M. vernalis,* and *M. autumnalis* produce chemicals that are trance-inducing. Egyptian papyri and tomb decorations show priest-shamans guiding the living and the dead, often accompanied by depictions of mandrake.

An Egyptian fresco from the fourteenth century B.C.E. shows Meriton, consort of Semenkhara (who is shown ill and leaning on a crutch), offering him two mandrakes and a water lily (N. caerulea). Meriton wears the sacred asp of Thoth on her forehead to indicate that she is a healer.

The Cairo collection of objects from Tutankhamen's tomb includes a jar showing a face of Hathor, Goddess of healing, wearing a necklace of water lilies and a mandrake fruit. Opioid residues were found in another of the jars. It is possible that blue water lily, mandrake, and opium could be conducive to the "little death," whereby a shaman leaves the physical body and communicates with beings on other planes.

The priestly castes are known to have invoked the trinity Ra-Horus-Osiris through the trance ecstasy brought on by the blue water lily and mandrake.

A chest from Tutankhamen's tomb, now in the Cairo Museum,

shows the ailing king leaning on a crutch. His wife Ankhesenamun offers him narcotic blue water lilies and opium-poppy fruits. She wears mandrake fruits on her head. Two female servants pick mandrake fruits for the couple.

A scene from the Amara period shows Akhenaton and Nefertiti in a similar mode. The same plants appear repeatedly in the imagery.

King Tutankhamen's personal jewelry included carnelian mandrakes hanging from white water lily flowers. Lapis lazuli and green glass were used in a motif of blue water lilies and the sacred scarab, image of the Sun God.*

The large, brown root of mandrake resembles a parsnip and can grow to three or four feet under ground. The root can be single or branched. The leaves are about a foot long, are sharp-pointed, and emerge directly from the root. They have an unpleasant smell and lie open upon the ground when mature. The bell-shaped purple and white flowers resemble primroses and develop on separate stalks three or four inches in height. The flowers are followed by a round fruit about the size of a small apple with an apple-like scent and a yellow-orange color.

Herbal Uses: The leaves are used in poultices for ulcers and in salves. The fresh root is emetic and purgative and the dried bark is emetic. This plant was used by the ancients as a soporific and an anesthetic for operations. CAUTION: *The root is fairly violent in its action and should be used only by persons with strong constitutions. It is not recommended for home use.*

Orthodox modern medicine teaches that the history of anesthesia began on October 16, 1846, at Massachusetts General Hospital when William Thomas Green Morton demonstrated the effectiveness of ether. Pliny, however, states in his *Historia Naturalis* that in C.E. 77, it was common to drink the juice of mandrake before operations of any kind, and that even the smell of it was sufficient to put some to sleep.

Dioscorides, a Greek surgeon in Nero's army who worked in the first century C.E., tells us in *De Materia Medica* that mandrake was used for insomnia, great pain, surgery, and cauterization. He also says that the scent of the apples could be enough to put someone to sleep.

---

* For an excellent overview of the Egyptian material, see William Emboden, "The Sacred Journey in Dynastic Egypt: Shamanistic Trance in the Context of the Narcotic Water Lily and the Mandrake," *Journal of Psychoactive Drugs*, Jan–March 1989, 21 (1).

In the Middle Ages, doctors used a *spongia somnifera* (soporific sponge) consisting of a fresh sea-sponge soaked in opium, hyoscyamine (henbane), mulberry juice, lettuce seed, hemlock, mandrake, and ivy and then dried in the sun. When it was needed for pain-killing, it was reconstituted with water and inhaled or dripped into the mouth. Fennel root or vinegar was the antidote used to revive the patient. Another formula for *spongia somnifera* was a combination of mandrake, poppy, hops, henbane, lactuca (wild lettuce), and mulberry. **CAUTION:** *Please do not try this at home. These herbs can be very dangerous, if not fatal, when ingested!*

Gilbertus, author of *Compendium Medicinae*, describes the use of a *confectio soporifera*, a wet towel soaked in various herbs, to cover the patient's face. The herbs were *Papaver somniferum* (poppy), the juice of which was obtained by making slits in the cortex of its seed-bearing capsule; *Hyoscyamus* (henbane), the narcotic and analgesic juice of which was derived from the leaf, seed, and flower; *Mandragora officinalis* (mandrake) juice, taken from roots, leaves, and apples; *Rubus* (blackberry), possibly added to flavor and color the other juices; *Senecio* (ivy), which was tonic and diuretic; *Cuscuta* (dodder, golden-thread), a close relative of the morning-glory family; and *Atropa belladonna*, the juice of whose leaf and root is narcotic and antispasmodic, stimulating to the respiration and the heart, and was used by the ancients as an antidote to opium poisoning. Gilbertus adds that the patient was awakened by inserting vinegar in the mouth.

As to more modern efforts, the *Medical Journal of Australia* reported in 1971 that the Ipswich General Hospital performed a double-blind trial of the hypnotic effects and side effects of "Mandrax" (mandrake in pill form) and found it "safe and satisfactory." No dangerous side effects were noted. In statistical analysis, its hypnotic potency was equal to two hundred milligrams of pentobarbitone sodium, and there was no statistically significant difference in the rate of onset of sleep relative to those taking pentobarbitone sodium.

Homeopathic Uses: Homeopaths use *Mandragora* for restless excitability, bodily weakness, epilepsy, hydrophobia, and a great desire for sleep.

Magical Uses: Mandrake is an herb of Mercury. It is said to protect against demoniacal possession (possibly because it was used by ancient herbalists to sedate manics). Old herbals recommend avoiding "contrary winds" while digging the root. The mandrake root is supposed to resemble the human form, male or female, and so has been used as a poppet.* Mandrake is placed on the mantle to bring prosperity and happiness to the home.

Mandrake is worn to attract love and repel diseases. The root is used in exorcism rites. To activate a dried root, one must display it prominently in the home for three days, after which it is soaked in water overnight. The water can then be sprinkled on entryways, windows, and people, and the root is ready for magical use.

To be able to travel without being noticed, have four masses said over the root, then carry it with you wrapped in black silk.

Mandrake was once held to be a cure for impotence and sterility. It was so respected as a magical aid that the first being to touch the root was said to die. Hence dogs were used to pull the root by enticing them with food after tying them to the herb. When the dog sprang for the food the root came out. (The dog later succumbed.)

CAUTION: *Mandrake should not be taken internally for magic-working.*

MEADOWSWEET, (QUEEN-OF-THE-MEADOW, BRIDEWORT, BRIDE OF THE MEADOW), *SPIRAEA ULMARIA* = *FILIPENDULA ULMARIA*

Parts Used: Root, flower, leaf.

A fragrant, white-flowered meadow herb with delicate leaves, dark green on top and whitish beneath, interruptedly pinnate with larger terminal leaflets, one to three inches long, and three- to five-lobed. The stems grow up to four feet in height and are sometimes purple. The flowers grow in clusters and have a strong, sweet smell. The leaves smell like almonds. The plant was once popular for strewing on floors.

Herbal Uses: Traditional herbalists simmered the flowers in wine to treat fevers and to cure depression. The fresh flower tops, taken in tea, promote sweating. Steep two tablespoons of the herb in one cup of boiled water for twenty minutes. Take one-quarter cup four times a day. A distilled water of the flowers makes an eyewash to treat burning and itching. Meadowsweet is a classic for diarrhea, especially valued for children. The leaf is added to wine to bring a "merry heart"—that is, to cure depression.

---

* A "poppet" is a magical effigy of a person. Sympathetic magic is used to direct spells by visualization, prayers, or even putting pins into the figure.

Meadowsweet contains methyl salicylate, making it a good herb for rheumatic complaints and flus. It is astringent and helps with indigestion. It has diuretic properties, which make it helpful in edema. The tea has been used for respiratory tract infections, gout, and arthritis. It can help bladder and kidney problems, epilepsy, and rabies.

The whole plant is used—roots, flowers, and leaves—with the root being more useful for fevers. To prepare the root, simmer two tablespoons of the dried root in one cup of water for twenty minutes. Take one cup a day. The leaf is placed in claret wine to enhance the taste, and it was at one time added to mead.

A related herb is *Spiraea filipendula* (dropwort), which has more delicate foliage than *S. ulmaria*, pink buds, and whiter, scentless blossoms. The root is decocted in white wine and honey or taken as powder to help the kidneys. It will also benefit the lungs when wheezing, shortness of breath, hoarseness, and thick phlegm are a problem. Simmer two teaspoons of the root in one cup white wine or water for twenty minutes. Take a quarter cup four times a day.

Homeopathic Uses: Homeopaths use *Spiraea ulmaria* (hardhack, meadowsweet) for persons who are "morbidly conscientious"—obsessive-compulsive—and for irritations of the urinary passages or the prostate gland, epilepsy, and hydrophobia. It is used for burning and pressure in the throat and a feeling of contraction that is not made worse by swallowing.

Magical Uses: According to Grieve, meadowsweet, water mint, and vervain were the three most sacred herbs of the Druids. An herb of Jupiter, meadowsweet is used in love spells. It is strewn to promote peace, and its scent cheers the heart.

Meadowsweet should be included in the bridal bouquet, for who is "Bride" but Brighid, patroness of the Druids and Bards!

MINT, *MENTHA SATIVA*, *MENTHA AQUATICA*

Part Used: The above-ground portions of the herb.

A very common herb in northern Europe and Russian Asia. It grows to eighteen inches in height with ovate, serrated, hairy leaves. The lilac-colored flowers cluster around the stem. Mint is found in shady moist locations such as river banks, stream beds, and marshes.

According to Grieve, mint was one of the Druids' most sacred plants.

Herbal Uses: The infusion of the herb has been used for diarrhea and as an emmenagogue (it brings down the menses). It is a classic for colds and influenza, especially when mixed with elder flowers—but be careful, as this remedy will make you sweat, and you must take care to keep well covered with blankets and woolens. Stomach flu is helped by a mint, elderflower, and yarrow combination in a standard infusion of two teaspoons per cup steeped for twenty minutes and taken in quarter-cup doses.

Mint is helpful in stomach complaints, but a strong infusion will be emetic (it makes one throw up). Mint tea eases colic and lifts depression. It relieves earaches when the fresh juice or a few drops of the essential oil are placed in the ear. A few drops of the oil in water, applied with a cloth, help burning and itching, heat prostration, and sunburn. Apply it directly to an itchy skin condition or sunburn. For heat prostration place the cool fomentation on the forehead and wrists.

Mint tea with honey soothes a sore throat. A classic cold remedy that will unblock the sinuses is two drops of essential oil of mint, two drops of essential oil of eucalyptus, and the juice of half a lemon in a cup of hot water. The mix is first inhaled and then drunk when warm.

CAUTION: *No more than two drops of the essential oils should be taken at any time, and no more than two cups a day of the above mixture. Larger doses can be toxic to the kidneys.*

Homeopathic Uses: Homeopaths use menthol (essential oil of *Mentha*) for neuritis, acute nasal catarrh, blocked eustachian tubes, pharyngitis, laryngitis, itching, and vulvar itching. Compresses of the oil and water relieve frontal headache, sinus pain, pain in the eyeballs, and mental confusion. Asthmatic conditions with headache and dry smoker's cough are benefited as well.

Magical Uses: Mint is placed in the home as a protective herb. It belongs to the sphere of Venus. Place it on the altar when you work healing spells. Mint brings easy travel, attracts prosperity, and is placed in the wallet to draw money.

MISTLETOE (BIRDLIME, GOLDEN BOUGH, HOLY WOOD), *VISCUM ALBUM*

Ad viscum Druidae cantare solebant
(The Druids are wont to sing to the mistletoe.)

Ovid

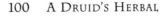

Parts Used: Twig and leaf.

Next to the oak tree, mistletoe is probably the plant most often associated with Druids. According to Pliny, the Druid priest or priestess would wear white robes to gather the herb, which was cut down on the sixth day of the moon or at Midsummer. A golden knife was used to gather the plant, and tremendous care was taken that it not touch the ground.* Two oxen were offered as a sacrifice for the harvest.

If the Druids failed to have visions of the plant for a long time or if it fell to earth for any reason, it was considered a bad omen.

Viscum album grows from northern Europe to northwest Africa and east to Asia and Japan. Different varieties are found on hardwood and softwood trees, which include apple (the most common), elm, oak, spruce, pine, and poplar. Druids considered that the mistletoe found on oak was the most potent and sacred.

The berries ripen in midwinter and have a further peculiarity in that the ripe berries, open flowers, green berries, and immature leaves can all be found on the same plant. Mistletoe does not adhere to the linear logic of most plants, with their budding, flowering, and seed production sequence. It also seems to ignore heliotropism and geotropism—it will grow upside down, sideways, or in any direction it "chooses." Another unique feature is that it germinates only in the light, unlike most plants, which require darkness to germinate. The flower buds form in May but do not open until February. The berries ripen the following winter. The entire process, from flower to fruit, can take almost two years! Even its name *mistl* (different) *tan* (twig) (from the Anglo-Saxon) reminds us of its peculiarities.

Mistletoe is a parasitic plant, generally spread by bird droppings. It forms a globular mass that can reach up to three feet in diameter. There are male plants and female plants, and both derive their water and minerals from the host tree and produce their own carbohydrates via photosynthesis.

Mistletoe seems to hold itself aloof from the rhythms and laws of the earthly seasons, and in this way parallels the illogical and uncontrolled growth of cancerous cells in the body. As early as 1961, laboratory studies demonstrated that mistletoe, along with other immunostimulant plants (such as eupatorium, astragalus, echinacea,

---

* The golden knife was probably a brass or bone sickle or knife which was gold-plated. Pure gold would be too soft for the harvesting of herbs.

acanthopanax, chamomilla, and sabal), inhibited tumors in mice. Fermented mistletoe taken from oak trees (*Iscador quercus*) was shown to stimulate the activity of killer cells and showed an especially strong effect on rat hepatomas (liver cancers). Unfermented mistletoe showed a strong effect on human leukemia (Molt 4) cells. Korean mistletoe (*Viscum coloratum*) was found to be more active in inhibiting the growth of leukemia L1210, especially when used fresh.

Mistletoe extracts have been shown to possess significant antitumor activity, not only against murine tumors but also in cases of Lewis' lung carcinoma, colon adenocarcinoma 38, and C3H adenocarcinomas of the breast. The extracts are not toxic and may be administered in high doses. Twenty drops four times a day is the average dose.

Herbal Uses: Mistletoe is rich in phosphorus, magnesium, potassium, and sulphur. Its proteins, polysaccharides, and fat substances are strongly tumor-inhibiting. Tumor-inhibiting bacteria have also been found in the plant. Mistletoe seems to increase killer cells (a type of immune cell), increase cell-mediated cytotoxic activities, and augment levels of granular lymphocytes.

Many nervous conditions such as convulsions, delirium, hysteria, neuralgia, urinary disorders, and heart conditions have benefited from the activity of mistletoe. It has also been used to temper the spasms of epilepsy. Mistletoe strengthens the heart and has been used as a heart tonic in cases of typhoid fever. It strengthens the glandular system and has helped with inflammation of the pancreas. It promotes hormonal balance when taken daily for six months.

Mistletoe is recommended for use after a stroke or when hardening of the arteries is suspected. It will stop pulmonary and intestinal bleeding caused by dysentery and typhoid. It helps to lower high blood pressure and raise low blood pressure, and it has been used to ease heavy menstrual flow, heart palpitations, hot flashes, and the anxiety associated with menopause. The fresh juice has been said to increase fertility in barren women.

Anthroposophical medicine has produced a remedy, Iscador, which is available from anthroposophical physicians and pharmacies. Otherwise, one can take the dried leaf powdered, or in tea, or as an alcohol tincture.

The green plant can be simmered using a standard concoction of two teaspoons of the herb per cup of water and taken in tablespoon doses several times a day. **CAUTION:** *The berries should not be used for*

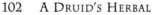

internal consumption! They are used in salves and washes for wounds. (See page 14 in chapter 2, "Herbal Basics," for directions on how to make salves.) Two ounces of leaves and twigs can be juiced, added to a half pint of spring water, and taken in tablespoon doses twice a day.

CAUTION: *Large doses have been known to induce convulsions in children—a clear revelation of its homeopathic nature.**

Homeopathic Uses: Homeopaths use *Viscum album* in low-potency or in a nonpotentized "mother tincture" for epileptic aura, petit mal seizures, heart conditions, asthma connected with gout or rheumatism, rheumatic deafness, chorea, metrorrhagia, and left-sided ovarian pain. Homeopaths recommend five to ten drops of tincture, several times a day, as a dose. Mistletoe is especially oriented to complaints on the left side of the body.

Magical Uses: Not quite herb, not quite tree, beyond the limitations of classification, freed from the restrictions of convention, and resembling a constellation of stars suspended in midair from the bough of a sacred tree—such is the "spirit" of this plant. It belongs to the in-between times of dusk and dawn, or the exact interval between two seasons. It is a gateway to something "other."

In Italy, there is an old tale of a radiantly beautiful fairy who appeared to a certain knight with the image of the crescent moon and the Holy Grail at her feet. In her hands she held a sprig of mistletoe. She told the knight that the mistletoe was what kept her eternally young and beautiful.

In the Edda of Scandinavia, a legend is recounted of Baldur—the "shining" god, who was troubled by dreams of his impending death. Frigg, the mother of the Gods, then asked all living beings to swear an oath not to kill him. However, she forgot the mistletoe. Loki, one of the old Gods and by tradition a troublemaker, tried to sabotage Frigg's efforts. He put a sprig of mistletoe into the hands of Hodur, who was blind, at a time when the Gods were making a game of throwing things at Baldur because it seemed that nothing could harm him. When Hodur hurled the mistletoe twig, Baldur was killed. The earth was plunged into mourning, as Baldur was the god who had given insight into the beauty of the shining spiritual world.

At the death of Baldur the world sank into spiritual darkness, a

---

* Homeopathic medicines are based on the observation that *similia similibus curentur*, or "like cures like." A substance that is capable of producing symptoms in a healthy individual will tend to *eliminate* those symptoms in someone who is ill.

"dark winter of the soul." (In considering the homeopathic dictum that "like cures like" or that "what causes disease can cure it," perhaps the story reveals how mistletoe, the agent of despair, is simultaneously the key to its remedy.)

Eventually, through the entreaties of all the Goddesses and Gods, Baldur was returned to life, and the light of the spiritual sun shone on earth once again.

Mistletoe was given into the keeping of the Goddess of love, and ever after people were enjoined to kiss under its branches.

Mistletoe is gathered on the sixth day of the moon or at Midsummer. It is carried as an herb of protection or placed where needed. Hung over a cradle it prevents the theft of a child by fairies. Amulets and jewelry can be made of its wood as talismans of protection and to speed healing. It will aid in hunting and in conception. Hang it in the bedroom to bring beautiful dreams and to unlock, through the dreams, the secrets of immortality. Add a few berries to the ritual cup at a handfasting, and hang it in the home to bring the blessings of the Goddess of love. CAUTION: *Never handle mistletoe where children might swallow fallen berries or leaves.*

Mistletoe is an excellent all-purpose magical herb. Its wood is a good choice for wands and ritual implements. Mistletoe is placed around a "Hand of Glory," a candle shaped like a hand that is burned to ward off thieves.

According to Virgil, Aeneas could go down to Tartarus only when he carried a sprig of mistletoe in his hand as protection. Mistletoe is reputed to protect the bearer from werewolves.

Mistletoe belongs to the sun and to Jupiter.

OAK (DUIR), *QUERCUS* SPP.

> Thanks invisible physician, for thy silent delicious medicine, thy day and night, thy waters and thy airs, the banks, the grass, the trees, and e'en the weeds
>
> **Walt Whitman, "The Oaks and I"**

Parts Used: Bark, leaf, acorn.

Oak is an open-branched tree that grows to ninety feet, with elliptical leaves having five to nine lobes, four to nine inches long and two to five inches wide. The leaves are purplish-red in the fall. The bark is light gray with shallow fissures and broad, loose, scaly plates. The acorns are three-eighths to one and a quarter inch long, eggshaped, and one-fourth enclosed by a cup. The bark and leaf are used medicinally.

While the white oak (*Quercus alba*) is the best for internal use, the bark of *Quercus robur*, the English oak, may also be used. A long-lived tree known to attain an age of a thousand years or more, it attains a height of eighty feet. Its leaves are two to five inches long and one and a quarter to two and a half inches wide, with six to fourteen shallow, rounded lobes. Two small ear-shaped lobes appear at the leaf base. The bark is dark gray with deep, irregular furrows. The acorns are five-eighths to one inch long, egg-shaped, and one-third enclosed by a cup.

The oak is so often associated with Druids that it could not be left out of this herbal. Of course, many other trees were sacred to the ancient Celts. Among them were birch, alder, elder, willow, holly, yew, hazel, hawthorn, ash, apple, and rowan. A full discussion of these is beyond the scope of this book; for more information please refer to my book *Tree Medicine, Tree Magic*. (Yew is not suited for home use, being highly poisonous).

Herbal Uses: Please see page 23 in "The Herbs of Samhain."

Magical Uses: The oak produces a wood for building that is incredibly strong yet pliable. It also makes the hottest blaze for heating the home. It has the ability to withstand lightning strikes, and it puts down roots that grow as deep as the tree is tall. All in all it symbolizes a powerful, balanced personality that is well prepared to stand the shock of sudden illumination or enlightenment.

We have plenty of archaeological evidence to support the tradition of the sanctity of the oak. Ancient Celtic oaken figures have been found at the source of the Seine. Oak wood was used for crypts in the Hallstatt and LaTene cultures, Celtic cultures distinguished by their unique styles of art. Sprays of oak, along with mistletoe, have been found in an ancient oak coffin.

According to Pliny, mistletoe was cut from an oak on the sixth day of the moon. A white-robed priest or priestess would climb the tree with a golden sickle and cut the herb, which dropped onto a white cloth. Two white bulls were sacrificed as part of the ritual.

The oak is portrayed as a supernatural tree in the story of Lleu, whose mother forbade him to marry an ordinary female. The magus Gwydion created the maiden Blodeuwedd of oak blossoms, broom, and meadowsweet for Lleu; but she betrayed her intended by taking a lover, who stabbed Lleu with a spear. Lleu then transformed himself into an eagle and flew to a magical oak tree to escape.

On Gaulish monuments, the Celtic thunder deity, Taranis, is often pictured in conjunction with oak trees. An oak, covered with mistletoe, is depicted on a silver cup discovered in Lyons. The pig, sacred to the Celts and a symbol of sexual and agricultural fertility and prowess in battle, relishes acorns.

The Goddess Brighid is associated with the oak tree. Saint Bridget of Kildare named her early monastic center "The Church of the Oak." It is well to remember that St. Bridget was born and raised as a Druidess before she took on the new Catholic faith.

A cross made of oak twigs (symbolic of the four sacred directions) and bound with a red thread is placed wherever one needs to ward off evil. The wood of oak can be carried for protection.

Acorns are used to increase fertility (of projects or ideas, or in matters of human reproduction) and to ward off pain. They are planted in the dark of the moon to bring financial prosperity. Symbolic of immortality, they are especially sacred to the Samhain (Halloween) season. Use them to decorate the altar in the fall.

Oak branches are made into wands and staves, after one asks the tree's permission (and gets an answer!). Do this in the waxing or full moon. A gift is left for the tree in exchange. Oak is burned in the Midsummer fire. A tree of the sun, its flames honor the Sun God at his height of power.

Oaks should be cut down in the waning moon. Be certain to give the tree spirit three day's warning so it can vacate and find a new home. Plant an acorn nearby to facilitate this process.

Beware of oaks during thunderstorms, as they tend to "draw the flash."

The oak is a tree of Jupiter.

SELAGO, *LYCOPODIUM SELAGO*, LINN.

Parts Used: Above-ground portions of the herb, and spores.

A member of the genus that also includes club moss and wolf's claw, selago was used magically and medicinally by Druids. The club mosses are found in North America, northern Europe, Asia, and the southern hemisphere. The plants are several inches in height and resemble moss. They creep by means of prostrate stems, which branch upward at intervals, with crowded, linear, simple leaves. Large two-valved spore cases produce the medicinally active spores.

Herbal Uses: While the whole plant was used by the ancients as a cathartic, the spores were used as a diuretic in edema, a drastic (a forceful agent of cure) in diarrhea and dysentery, a nervine for rabies and spasms, a mild laxative in cases of gout and scurvy, and a corroborant (strengthening agent) for rheumatism. The dose is ten to sixty grains of the spores.

The spores also make a dusting powder for skin diseases and diaper rash.

The herb, *L. selago*, is emetic (induces vomiting) and cathartic (induces defecation) in small doses.

CAUTION: *Selago can be an active narcotic poison when overused.* For this reason it is probably better to use only the spores, which are non-toxic. The whole plant can be used externally, however, as a counterirritant—made into a poultice, it will keep blisters open and kill lice. See page 15 for instructions in how to make a poultice.

Native Americans used the spores of *Lycopodium* to stop nosebleeds and to stop the bleeding of wounds. The spores were also used to absorb fluids from various injuries.

Homeopathic Uses: Homeopaths use *Lycopodium* for urinary and digestive disturbances, especially when malnutrition or liver involvement is suspected. Yellowish spots on the skin, a tendency to catarrh, and, in children, a sickly disposition in general are characteristic indications. Symptoms tend to run from right to left and are worse on the right side of the body. Between 4:00 and 8:00 P.M. is the worst time for all symptoms. The patient craves warm drinks; has poor circulation, cold extremities, and pains that come and go; and tends to be sensitive to noise and odors. Mentally, there is melancholy, apprehension, and a loss of self-confidence.

Homeopathic *Lycopodium* can be safely used internally (homeopathic medicines are extremely dilute).

Magical Uses: The spores of *Lycopodium* are highly flammable. Magicians once used them to create "lightning flashes" and other pyrotechnics as needed. These effects were originally intended as a form of sympathetic magic—of evocation by emulation—not simply (or deceptively) as stage effects.

Druids respected the plant to such a degree that it was gathered only under strict ritual guidelines. One of the Ovates would dress in white, bathe both feet in free-running water and offer a sacrifice of bread and spirits, and then with white robe wrapped around the right hand, using a brass hook,* would dig up the plant by the roots. The herb was immediately covered by a white cloth.

When properly gathered, the herb becomes a charm of power and protection. Wear it, add it to incense, and use it to commune with the Gods and Goddesses.

SELF-HEAL (ALL-HEAL, HEART-OF-THE-EARTH), *PRUNELLA VULGARIS*

Self-Heal whereby when you are hurt, you may heal yourself.

Nicholas Culpeper

Part Used: Above-ground portions of the herb.

A member of the Labiatae family, this plant is easily found in grassy meadows at the edges of woods in Europe and America. It grows from one to three feet in height and has slightly hairy, square stems. The petioled opposite leaves are oblong-lanceolate, and the tiny, two-lipped, purple flowers are arranged in tiers composed of rings of six to twelve stalkless blossoms.

Herbal Uses: The name *Prunella* is from the German *Brunellen*, given to the herb because it cures *die Breuen* or "trench mouth," a bacterial infection of the mucous lining of the mouth and throat. This condition is often developed by soldiers who spend much time in garrisons. Mixed with honey in a simple infusion, it is also excellent for sore throats. Steep two teaspoons of the herb in one cup of boiled water for twenty minutes. The dose is one-fourth cup, four times a day.

Self-heal is applied in poultices and salves to external ulcers and wounds and is taken as a tea to heal internal injuries and to recover from surgery. See pages 14 and 15 for the instructions for making poultices and salves.

As an astringent, the herb is helpful for diarrhea when taken as a tea and for hemorrhages when used both internally and externally. It has been used to lower fevers and in hepatitis, jaundice, high blood

---

* Druids of highest rank customarily carried a gold-covered brass sickle to use in the gathering of sacred plant medicines.

pressure, and edema. The Chinese value it for its antitumor properties.

In 1988, it was reported that *Prunella vulgaris* and *Selaginella doederleinii* (a Lycopodium) demonstrated an antimutagenic effect of over fifty percent in salmonella bacteria that had been exposed to picrolonic acid or benzopyrene. *Prunella vulgaris* was found to contain antimutagenic factors against both directly and indirectly induced mutations.[*]

In another 1989 study, an anti-HIV compound was isolated from infusions of *P. vulgaris*.[†] Chang and Yeung had reported in 1988 that water infusions of *P. vulgaris* and other herbs used in Chinese medicine inhibited the in vitro growth of HIV virus. (*Prunella* had long been known to traditional Chinese herbalists as an antiinfective agent).

Homeopathic Uses: Homeopaths use *Prunella* primarily for colitis.

Magical Uses: Druids gathered self-heal in a manner similar to that used for vervain (*Verbena officinalis*). It was to be picked when the Dog Star was rising, at night, during the dark of the moon. It was dug up by the roots with the Druid's golden sickle and then held aloft in the left hand. After prayers of thanksgiving were said, the flowers, leaves, and stalks were separated for drying.

Place self-heal on the altar when working healing magic. And be sure to leave a gift for the Earth to compensate her for her loss when you pick this precious herb.

Self-heal is an herb of Venus.

VERVAIN (ENCHANTER'S HERB, HERB OF GRACE), *VERBENA OFFICINALIS*

Part Used: Above-ground portions of the herb.

A perennial herb found in Europe, North Africa, China, and Japan. (*Verbena hastata*, the blue vervain, is a native of the Americas.) The plant has opposite leaves with toothed lobes; a stiff, quadrangular stem; and white or lilac flowers that appear from June to October. The flowers grow on slender spikes and are without scent.

Herbal Uses: "Vervain" is a derivative of the Celtic *fer* (to drive away)

---

[*] Huei Lee and Jung-Yaw Lin, *Mutation Research*.
[†] K. M. Smith, H. D. Tabba, and R. S. Chang, *Antiviral Research*.

and *faen* (stone), given to it because of its ability to purge calculi (gravel) from the bladder. A tea of the herb helps to increase breast milk and is helpful in lowering fever, especially of the intermittent type. It will benefit eczema and other skin eruptions, as it is a kidney and liver cleanser. Jaundice, whooping cough, edema, mastitis, and headaches fall under its sphere. To make the tea, steep one tablespoon of the herb per cup of water for twenty minutes. For tincture, follow the instructions given on page 15 and take twenty to forty drops in water as needed.

Externally, vervain is used in poultices for ear infections, rheumatism and wounds.

Vervain is an emmenagogue (brings down the menses) and soothes the nerves. It is reputed to have aphrodisiac properties. It is a powerful lymphatic detoxifier and has a cleansing effect on the female organs.

Blue vervain (*Verbena hastata*), the American variety, is a natural tranquilizer and is helpful with colds and fevers, especially when the upper respiratory tract is involved. It will eliminate intestinal worms and is used externally for wounds. It is distinguished from the European vervain by its deeper blue flowers and denser, bristly flower spikes.

Blue vervain is also prepared in a standard infusion or tinctured in alcohol.

Homeopathic Uses: Homeopaths use *Verbena* (blue vervain) for conditions involving the skin and the nervous system. The tincture has been used as a remedy for poison oak. Epilepsy, insomnia, constipation, and mental exhaustion are helped by it. In cases involving epilepsy, the tincture should be taken for prolonged periods of time.

Magical Uses: Vervain is a profoundly magical herb belonging to the sphere of Venus. Roman priests and priestesses used it as an altar plant—it was tied in bundles and used to ritually "sweep" and purify the altar. Druids placed it in water that was sprinkled on worshipers as a blessing.

Vervain was picked at the rising of the Dog Star, at the dark of the moon, just before flowering. It was taken from the earth with the sacred sickle and raised aloft in the left hand. After prayers of thanksgiving were spoken, the Druid or Druidess left a gift of honey to recompense the Earth for her loss.

Vervain was once infused in wine and worn on the body to ward off the stings of insects and serpents. It is used in the bath as a protection from enchantments and to make dreams come true.

Wearing or bathing in vervain places one under the influence of Diana. After washing your hands in the infusion, it will be possible to engender love in the one you touch.

To dispel fears, light a candle daily and surround it with vervain. Speak aloud a prayer to the Gods and Goddesses asking for release from your fear. Do this as long as necessary.

On the night of the full moon, go outside with a chalice filled with water, vervain, and salt. Take also a candle and a piece of petrified wood. Dip the stone into the water mixture and then pass it through the candle flame. Touch the stone to your feet, hands, shoulders, and head. As you do this ask for the blessings of youth and beauty. Repeat the process seven times.

Vervain is worn as a crown during Druidic initiatory rites and as a protection for those who are working magic. It is sprinkled throughout the home or ritual area and burned as incense as a protection and to bring peace. Keep some in the bedroom to bring tranquil dreams. Keep it in the home to attract wealth and to keep plants healthy. Sprinkle some on the garden as an offering to the elementals and other nature spirits. Drinking the juice of fresh vervain is said to cut sexual desire. Burn it to banish the pangs of unrequited love.

Vervain is worn to recover stolen articles. Tucked into a child's cradle, the plant brings joy and a lively intellect.

WATER HOREHOUND (GYPSYWEED), *LYCOPUS EUROPAEUS*

Part Used: Above-ground portions of the herb.

A plant that was once used to dye wool black, water horehound flowers by stream banks throughout Europe from July to September. It attains a height of about two feet and has pointed, toothed leaves and small, pinkish flowers that grow in the axils of the higher leaves.

Herbal Uses: This plant was used as an astringent and as a sedative. Because little information is available regarding its use, it may be best understood through an examination of a related plant, *Lycopus virginicus*, which is common in the United States. Known as bugleweed, it has a perennial, creeping root, a quadrangular square stem, and attains a height of up to twenty-four inches. It bears opposite leaves, which are lanceolate and toothed, the lower leaves being more wedge-shaped. The flowers grow in the leaf axils with four lobed, purplish corollas.

As a sedative, astringent, and mild narcotic, bugleweed has been used to soothe coughs and bleeding from the lungs (as from tuberculosis). It is best when used fresh or freshly tinctured in alcohol, not dried. The fresh herb is steeped using two teaspoons of herb per cup of water for twenty minutes. For the tincture, follow the general directions given on page 15. The dose is ten to thirty drops, three or four times a day.

A Chinese species (*L. lucidus*) also grows in marshy and damp environments and is used for menstrual and urinary problems (it is emmenagogic and diuretic). It is used externally in liniments for cardiac problems but should be avoided in pregnancy.

In vivo research (live animal studies) in 1985 has shown that water horehound, bugleweed, lemon balm (*Melissa officinalis*), and stoneseed (*Lithospermum officinalis*) exhibit antithyrotropic activity and inhibit the biological activity of Grave's disease, a condition that involves an enlarged thyroid, rapid pulse, and increased metabolism. (These plants had been used for untold generations by traditional herbalists to treat hyperthyroidism.)*

Homeopathic Uses: Homeopaths use *Lycopus virginicus* to lower blood pressure and for valvular heart disease, heart palpitations, passive hemorrhages, and toxic goiter. Urinary symptoms for which it is beneficial include a profuse quantity of watery urine, the sensation of a distended bladder even when empty, and testicular pain. It has been found useful in diabetes. Indications include wakefulness and "morbid vigilance" that prevents sleep.

Magical Uses: The flowers and leaves of water horehound and bugleweed are offered to deities in the form of incense and garlands.

WILD BASIL, *CALAMINTHA CLINOPODIUM*

Part Used: Above-ground portions of the herb.

This wild variety of basil is common in England and Scotland and rare in Ireland. The plant attains a height of about a foot and has opposite egg-shaped leaves on a square stem. The stem and leaves are

---

* Auf'mkolk, Ingbar, Kubota, Amir, and Ingbar, *Endocrinology* 1985 May 116 (5), pp. 1687-93.

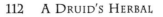

slightly hairy. The flowers are pink and spring from the bases of the leaf stalks. Wild basil favors dry hedges in higher elevations.

Herbal Uses: According to Grieve, wild basil is rich in aromatic oils and resembles thyme and calamint in its action.

As information on the ancient uses of wild basil is scarce, an overview of calamint, thyme, and basil thyme will be given here as an aid to understanding the action of wild basil.

Calamint (*Calamintha ascendens* = *Melissa calaminta*) grows to about a foot in height, with downy, square stems and opposite leaves. The flowers are light purple. It has a minty smell.

Culpeper warns us that women should use the plant cautiously, as it has a strong effect on the female reproductive system. The herb was once used to bring on menstruation and to ease cramps. Traditionally, it was said to "hinder" conception in women. Equal parts of wild thyme, basil thyme, wild basil, calamint, and garden thyme are prepared in a standard infusion of two teaspoons per cup of water steeped for twenty minutes and taken in quarter-cup doses four times a day. Calamint was used as a poultice to ease the pains of sciatica, (please see page 15 for directions on how to make a poultice). The tea was used to strengthen the stomach and to help with gas and colic.

Calamint has psychic effects as well. It has been used to calm hysteria, cure melancholy, and bring gladness to the heart.

Calamint is useful in jaundice, being a liver and spleen cleanser. Externally, it is used in poultices for bruises. It is used in syrups for coughs and colds as an expectorant.

Garden thyme (*Thymus vulgaris*), a woody-stalked, low-growing shrubby plant, has tiny, pink flowers, which grow in clusters at the stem tips. The leaves are about one-eighth inch long, narrow, and paired.

Thyme is known primarily as a lung cleanser and an herb to dry up moist lung conditions. Thyme tea is excellent for babies with moist coughs.

It is used to help expel the afterbirth and also as a wound herb, because of its antiseptic properties. Failing eyes and sciatica benefit from its external use as a poultice. Internally, it eases headaches, gas, colic, and hangovers. Combine thyme and rosemary for migraine headaches.

Wild thyme (*Thymus serpyllum*) is the indigenous thyme of northern Europe. It is a small plant, often found in dense clusters growing in exposed areas. In protected areas, it sends out stalks of a foot or so in height. The stems are woody and reddish-brown; the leaves are opposite and about one-eighth inch wide, with hairs at the base and prominent veins on the undersurface. The flowers are reddish purple and form clusters at the tips of the stems.

Headaches, nervous conditions, nightmares, hangovers, dizziness, and intestinal gas are treated with this herb. Not quite as powerful as garden thyme, it helps with sore throats and coughs. Vinegar of thyme is rubbed on the temples to relieve headache.

Homeopaths use *Thymus serpyllum* in tincture for children's chest complaints, asthma of the nervous type, and whooping cough with ringing in the ears and a burning sore throat.

Basil thyme (*Calamintha acinos*) is a classic of traditional herbalism. While common in England, it is rare in Scotland and Ireland. It is a bushy plant with branching stems that grow about six to eight inches. The leaves are one-quarter to one-half inch long, egg-shaped, and slightly hairy, with prominent veins on the undersides. The flowers are bluish-purple and white, about one-half inch long and growing on the stem tips.

Basil thyme was administered as a tea to those who were bitten by snakes. The fresh herb was used as a poultice to treat bruises and burned or strewn to repel snakes. It was used as a bath additive for children to strengthen and calm the nerves. The oil has been used to ease toothache (use one drop on a bit of cotton) and as an external rub for sciatica and neuralgia.

By studying the virtues of these herbs, we can come close to an understanding of how the ancient Druids may have used wild basil. Basically known for its stomachic, styptic, and emmenagogic properties, it was also used to make a yellow and a brown dye.

Magical Uses: Basil is a traditional herb of protection under the dominion of Mars. It is soaked in water for three days and sprinkled in entrance ways to repel thieves. It will attract customers to a place of business. Basil leaves left exposed in a room will dispel melancholy and bring joy. It is rubbed on the skin or carried for protection in crowds.

Basil is a classic herb for couples, as it tends to mend quarrels. Add it to power bundles and love spells. Sprinkle it over a sleeping loved one to ensure his or her fidelity.

Use basil in the ritual bath and in incense for purification. It brings courage and eases transitions in rites of initiation. Basil is a holy herb of the Hindu tradition, sacred to Vishnu.

Thyme is a house blessing herb and is used as incense to encourage health. It brings vitality and strength to one who carries it while walking. A classic for healing spells, it is placed near the bed to ward off nightmares. Wear the herb to enhance psychic powers.

Thyme was used by the Greeks to purify their temples. It is burned to purify a ritual space and used in the ritual bath to wash away the sorrows of the past. It is sacred to Venus.

Once again, we must look to the uses of basil and thyme to gain a sense of how the ancient Druids may have used wild basil for magical purposes. According to one source, the plant was used by Druids as a ritual offering to the gods.

WOAD, *ISATIS TINCTORIA*

Part Used: Leaf.

From southern and western Europe to Sweden and west Asia, woad (from the Anglo-Saxon *Wad*) was once commonly used as a dye. Julius Caesar records that the British natives used it to paint their bodies blue when they went naked to their rituals.

The plant grows to about three feet in height and has long, bluish-green leaves that branch out, small yellow flowers, and black seeds. It flowers from June to September and produces a single white root.

Herbal Uses: According to Culpeper, woad was used to poultice the area of the spleen when there was pain in that region. A poultice is generally made by mashing the green herb or soaking the dried herb in hot water until soft and adding slippery elm powder or buckwheat flower to make a paste. Woad was simmered into salves for weeping ulcers and to stop bleeding. Please see pages 14 and 15 for instructions on the making of poultices and salves.

The leaf produces a blue color in wool that has been mordanted with alum and potassium carbonate.

Now, why would our ancestors paint themselves blue? This custom may have been merely symbolic or of religious significance—or perhaps it had a more practical application. I am inclined to think that several thousand years ago folks were about as intelligent as they are today and that they tended to nurture customs that had survival value.

According to one scienfific study, tryptanthrin—an antimicrobial substance that is effective against dermatophytes (funguses that cause skin diseases such as ringworm)—has been isolated from *Polygonum tinctorium*, a Japanese variety of indigo, and from *Isatis tinctoria*, woad.*

Japanese indigo is a plant used to dye cloth blue, and it is antifungal. It has traditionally been used to cure *T. mentagrophytes*, athletes' foot. Woad also tests positive for antifungal activity against *T. mentagrophytes*. While there is no record or evidence of its use as an antifungal, it could easily have been used as one! (Imagine what life was like in the damp, misty isles of northern Europe, and you can speculate on how useful this practice of painting the body with woad must have been.)

Magical Uses: Woad belongs to Mars and Jupiter. I could find no reference for the magical use of woad other than that of Julius Caesar. Why not honor the memory of the ancient Celts and Picts by tattooing your arms, legs, face, or body with the dye? The ancients would have cut magical designs into their bodies and rubbed in the blue coloring. You may simply prefer to paint it on for ceremonial purposes.

THE SCIENTIFIC EVIDENCE

Bog studies using core samples have provided evidence to show which plants were native to Ireland before the Roman and Christian periods in Europe. The following lists are from *The Flora and Vegetation of Britain* by Harley and Lewis.

These pollen counts were taken from a bog in the county Antrim, Northern Ireland.

MESOLITHIC AND NEOLITHIC

Filicales	ferns
Polypodium	ferns
Osmunda	ferns
Lycopodium	club moss
Isoetes	(Merlin's) quillwort

---

* G. Honda, J. Tosirisuk, *Planta Medica*.

Myriophyllum	water weed
Nymaphaea	water lily
Potamogeton	floating round plant
Polyganum amphibium	water knotweed
Typhales	cat tails
Lysimachia	fireweed, loosestrife
Filipendula	meadowsweet
Myrica	bayberry
Cyperaceae	sedges
Umbellifera	miscellaneous apiaceae
Rosaceae	roses
Cruciferae	cabbages, etc.
Compositae	daisies
Caryophyllaceae	carnation
Ericaceae	heather
Pteridium	bracken
Artemisia	mugwort
Plantago lanceolata	plantain
Gramineae	grass
Tilia	lime (linden)
Hedera	ivy
Fraxinus	ash
Corylus	hazel
Salix	willow
Alnus	alder
Quercus	oak
Ulmus	elm
Pinus	pine
Betula	birch

MESOLITHIC

Menyanthes	buckbean
Helianthinum	sunflowers
Galium	cleavers
Malus	apple
Ranunculus	buttercups
Achillea	yarrow
Taraxacum	dandelion
Ilex	holly

Taxus	yew
Leucoizum	summer snow
Pedicularis	lousewort
Digitalis	foxglove
Scrofularia	figwort
Cornus	dogwood
Viburnum	miscellaneous
Ligustrum	privet
Populus	poplar
Juniperus	juniper

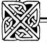

CHAPTER 12

Herbal Alchemy and the Planets

But if he (the physician) does not know the world, nor the elements or the firmament, how should he discover the nature of man, who is everything that is in heaven and on earth, indeed, who is himself heaven and earth, air and water?

Paracelsus

The light of nature in man comes from the stars.

Paracelsus

Penetrating into the earth, I sustain all creatures by My strength; by becoming the moon full of juices, I nourish all plants.

Bhagavad Gita 15:13

A traditional concern of the Druid is for the relationship between the matter and forces of the Earth and the matter and forces of the celestial sphere. After all, the Earth and every living thing on her shores and in her waters originated in the stars, born from the coagulation of star gases and warmed and fed by nourishing stellar winds.

Ancient herbalists classified herbs by their planetary affiliations. When studying these affiliations, we are actually examining the vibrations inherent in the plant that resemble its planetary ruler. By ingesting these plants we partake of the celestial intelligence, consciousness, knowledge, and power of that particular planetary sphere.

The knowledge of the usefulness of plants on four levels—mental, physical, emotional, and spiritual—is the basis of true alchemy whereby our body's subtle energies are gradually transmuted into the pure gold of cosmic wisdom, unconditional love, and infinite power.

The consciousness of the herbalist is an important factor in the preparation of the remedy. One may choose to imagine a color surrounding the herbal preparation, or one can bless it with a prayer. Those who work with color healing may wish to project a healing color onto the remedy that will act to enhance its intended effect.

Here are some examples of the spiritual nature of color: red for vitality; violet for deep cleansing and the transmutation of negative energies; blue for deep relaxation, forgiveness, protection, and the opening of blocked or "inflamed" channels; pink for the qualities of unconditional love and to soothe a broken heart; emerald green for its balancing qualities; purple to enhance personal mastery; and white for its all-encompassing healing nature. Use your intuition to select an appropriate color aura for your herbs.

Select these herbs as you would any therapeutic tool—the aim is to heal the individual from within his or her innermost being. Mental and spiritual harmony will result in emotional balance, which in turn acts to free the vital forces of the body. Once strengthened and free-flowing, the vital forces can move to wherever they are needed and accomplish their natural function: perfect health on all levels of being.

SUN-RULED PLANTS

Solar herbs will tend to be orange, reddish-orange, and yellow.

Strong magnetic fields, particle-rich solar winds, and the life-nourishing warmth of the sun sustain all forms of life on our planet. The solar metals, gold and copper,* reflect the light, warmth, and incredible vitality of our closest star.

The body systems ruled by solar energies are the heart, circulation, spine, vital force and heat of the body, thymus gland, pons varolii, and eyes. The sun also rules the spleen, which transforms energies and sends them on to the solar plexus, the center of the *qi*, or vital force. From there the energies are radiated to the whole system.

Diseases associated with the sun are constitutional, organic, and

---

* Copper is a solar metal in East Indian systems of thought.

structural. The chrysolith and the ruby will help attract solar energy to the body.

On the psychic plane, the sun is associated with positive ego strength. It enhances the personal will so that the individual finds the strength to manifest her or his divine purpose. Inferiority complexes are overcome, and the quality of generosity is enhanced in the personality. Ambition, courage, dignity, and self-reliance are fostered by these plants. Managerial skills and a sense of personal authority are bolstered.

The sun represents the divine creative principle. It can counteract apathy and help propel one out of an unproductive period.

Some specific herbs of the sun are given here.

For the heart: butterbur, mistletoe, borage, motherwort.

For vitality: grapes.

HERBS OF THE SUN

almond (with Jupiter)
angelica (with Venus)
ash tree (with Jupiter)
bay tree
bergamot
burnet
butterbur
calamus
centaury (also lesser centaury)
chamomile
celandine (greater) (with Jupiter)
cinnamon
cinquefoil
clove
dittany
elecampane
eyebright
feverfew
gentian (with Jupiter and Mars)
ginger
grapevine (with Jupiter)

ground ivy (with Venus)
heart trefoil
honewort
juniper bush (with Jupiter and Mercury)
laurel (with Jupiter)
lemon balm (with Jupiter)
lemon tree
lovage
marigold
male peony
marshmallow (with Jupiter and Venus)
meadow rue
mistletoe (with Jupiter and Moon)
mustards (white and black) (with Mars)
olive tree (with Jupiter)
orange tree
peony
passionflower

pepper (white and black)
pimpernel
plantain (with Mars)
ribwort (with Mars)
rice
rosemary
rue
saffron
scarlet pimpernel (with Jupiter)
St. John's wort
St. Peter's wort
storax tree
strawberry (with Jupiter)
sundew
sunflower
thyme (with Venus)
tormentil
turnsole
viper's bugloss
walnut tree (with Mercury)
zeodary

MOON-RULED PLANTS

Lunar herbs tend to have white or yellow flowers and soft, juicy leaves, and to live in or near water.

The moon is intimately connected with waters and fluids of all kinds. High tide and low tide are governed by the position of the moon. At full moon, hemorrhages are more frequent and harder to control, nocturnal activities of all kinds pick up, and the number of births increases.

Physiologically the moon rules the stomach and esophagus, ovaries, womb, and breasts. All fluid secretions of the body and associated organs are affected by lunar activity: menstruation, blood, urinary bladder, cerebellum, pancreas.

The moon rules the fluids in the eyes, brain, glands, libido, thyroid, tonsils, and tears. Lunar diseases are those associated with periodicity. Irregular menstruation, epilepsy, somnambulism, and hysteria are aggravated.

In the psychic realm, moon-ruled plants have an affinity for the subconscious mind. Hypnosis and autohypnosis can be more easily effected, and ingrained habits are more easily broken.

Lunar herbs facilitate past-life recall and channeling skills. Otherwise inexplicable habits and addictions may be removed or altered when past-life traumas are brought to conscious awareness. Astral forms and functions come closer to awareness with the use of these herbs. Simultaneously, they promote a resurgence of interest in matters of the home and common domestic details.

Lunar herbs help one to unwind and gain an appreciation for the simple gifts of life. They impart grace to the gait and help put one in tune with others. They increase sensitivity and imagination and put one into the rhythm of the lifestream.

Silver, moonstone, pearls, and amber best transmit the lunar forces. The plant world in general is under the influence of the moon.

Some specific herbs of the moon are given here.

For the blood: adder's tongue, wintergreen (*Pyrola minor*), loosestrife, white roses, cleavers, lettuce.

For the lymph: cleavers, chickweed, wild poppy.

For the hormones: saxifrage.

For the stomach: clary, wild poppy, cucumber, orpine, white roses, dog rose.

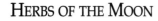

HERBS OF THE MOON

adder's tongue
acanthus
arrach
arrowhead
atriplex (orache)
banana
brankursine
brassicae
cabbage
caltrops
chickweed
clary
cleavers
colewort
coralwort
corn poppy (with Saturn)
cucumber
cuckoo flower
daisy (bellis)
dog-tooth violet
duckweed
fleur-de-lys
faverel (woolly)
fluetin

gourds
hawkweed (mouse ear)
hyssop
iris (with Saturn)
lady's smock
lettuce
lily (white garden)
loosestrife
mango
mercury (French)
melons
moonwort
moneywort
monk's pepper
mouse ear
nutmeg
opium poppy (with Saturn)
orpine
orris root
papaya
pearlwort
pearl trefoil
periwinkle
poppy (white or opium)

poppy (wild)
privet
pumpkin
purslane
pelitory of Spain
rattle grass
rose (dog)
rose (white)
saxifrage (great burnet)
saxifrage (small burnet)
sedum
seaweed
speedwell
soldier (common water)
stonecrop
sweet flag
turmeric
wallflower (common)
water chestnut
watercress
water lily
water violet
wild lettuce
willow tree
wintergreen

MERCURY-RULED PLANTS

Mercurial plants tend to have fine or highly divided leaves. Mercury is the planet closest to the great, central sun. To the Egyptians, Thoth, also known as Hermes Trismegistus, reflected the mercurial essence. Thoth was said to have invented written and spoken language. He was also patron of the art of medicine.

Mercury rules the intellect, speech, writing, and communication as well as the nervous system and its fluids, ears, hearing, tongue, vocal cords, bronchii, lungs, and thyroid. In the brain, Mercury rules the pons, which unites the Sun-ruled cerebrum with the Moon-ruled cerebellum. The diseases ruled by Mercury are associated with the organs governed by whatever zodiacal signs the planet is transiting.

Quicksilver, topaz, opal, tourmaline, peridot, and emerald carry the energies of Mercury.

The use of the herbs and stones of Mercury brings keenness, versatility, and wit, as Mercury enhances the ability to make associations. Writers and speakers will find their talents increased. Mixed with solar and lunar herbs, these plants engender a harmony of spirit that facilitates contact with the *Akasha* (the great etheric record of all that ever has been or will be over time).

Those who use the power of the spoken word to aid in manifestation will find their practice improved. Mixed with lunar herbs, psychic receptivity is enhanced. Mixed with solar herbs, telepathic sending abilities are strengthened.

These plants facilitate linkage between the macrocosm and the microcosm, the "as above" and the "so below." They promote contacts with different spheres and improve mediumship.

Some specific herbs of Mercury are given here.

For the nerves: marjoram, valerian, summer savory.

For the brain: dill, lavender, lily of the valley.

For the lungs: elecampane, fennel, horehound, licorice, maidenhair, pellitory-of-the-wall, flaxseed oil, fenugreek, summer savory, valerian.

For the sight: caraway, white horehound, lily of the valley, upright water parsnip.

Herbs of Mercury

acacia	coltsfoot	goat's rue
agaric	cubeb pepper	good Henry
amara dulcis	digitalis (with Venus	hazelnut
anise	and Saturn)	honeysuckle
azalea	dill	hop trefoil (hopclover)
bittersweet	dog's Mercury	horehound
bryony	elecampane	hound's tongue (with
buckbean	fennel	Jupiter)
calamint (wild basil)	fennel flower	lavender (with Sun and
caraway	fenugreek	Jupiter)
carrot	flax	lavender cotton
celery	fern (brake or bracken)	lily of the valley
chicory (endive) (with	garlic	licorice
Jupiter)	germander	maidenhair

mandrake (with moon and Saturn)	oregano	savory (summer)
	parsley	(winter)
mercury (annual and perennial)	parsnip	scabious
	pellitory of Spain	smallage
mulberry tree	pellitory-of-the-wall	southernwood
mushroom	pomegranate tree	spignel (broad leaved)
myrtle tree	rampion (sheep's)	trefoil
nailwort	sauce-alone (common garlic cress)	valerian
nux vomica		wormwood (with Venus)
oat (with Jupiter)		

VENUS-RULED PLANTS

The herbs of Venus have extraordinarily beautiful flowers and tend to have red fruits.

Venus appears to us as the morning and evening star. In Babylon, Greece, and Rome, the planet was regarded as the female embodiment of sexual love. In her guise as Ishtar, Ashtaroth, Aphrodite, or Venus, she could influence both heterosexual and homosexual unions. In other cultures—Egyptian, Mayan, Phoenician, Hebrew, and Indian—Venus was seen as male. Teacher, physician, and bestower of the elixir of immortality, Venus was closely associated with the alchemical arts.

Venus rules the internal sexual organs as well as the umbilical cord, nose, sense of smell, neck, palate, and spine. Venus influences the harmony between the various body systems, cell transformation and growth, the tone of the tissues, the complexion, and the appearance of the face. The abdomen, kidney, parathyroid glands (which influence calcium metabolism), thymus, and breasts fall under Venus' dominion.

All matters of appetite, such as overindulgence that leads to disease, are under Venus, as are the chyle in the intestines, the diuretic and emetic processes, the veins of the stomach, and all internal secretions. Venus does not in itself promote disease. A bad configuration with other planets results in diseases of the kidneys, uterus, and sex organs.

Copper, pink coral, jade, and diamonds bring the energies of Venus to the aspirant. The herbs and minerals of Venus act to increase personal magnetism and refine the senses. Musicians, artists, actors, and those who seek to mediate between the classes and interest groups of society will find their work enhanced. Venus promotes affection, amiability, and style.

Venus bestows greater sensitivity to astral influences, bringing inspiration and personal charm. The subtle vibrations of inner beauty are enhanced. Harmony and balance in one's personal life and in dealings with others will be increased, as will contact with the subtle forces of nature. Venus opens consciousness to the secrets of the plant kingdom, and contact with the ancient nature religions is strengthened.

Some specific herbs of Venus are given here.

For the kidneys: eryngo, kidney wort, french beans, feverfew, mint, yarrow, burdock, plantain, common sorrel, strawberries.

For the bladder: beans, elderberries, eryngo, common mallow, marshmallow, peach tree leaves, violet, plantain (buck'shorn), wood sorrel.

For the testes: marshmallow, beans, thyme.

For the throat: thyme, coltsfoot, cowslip, marshmallow.

For the ovaries: lady's mantle, mint, thyme, mugwort, pennyroyal.

For the veins: lady's mantle, damask rose, self-heal, wood sorrel.

HERBS OF VENUS

alder
alkanet
alehoof
alder (black)
apple (with the Sun)
artichoke
archangel
archangel bean
beans (broad) (with the Moon)
beans (French)
birch tree
bishop's weed
blackberry
blites
bramble
bugle
burdock
catmint

cherry tree
chestnut (with Jupiter)
chickpea
coltsfoot
columbine
cotyledon (navelwort)
cowslip
crab's claw
crosswort
cudweed
daffodil
daisy
devil's bit
digitalis (with Mercury and Saturn)
dittander (karse)
dittany of Crete
dittany (white)
dropwort

dyer's alkanet
elder (with Saturn and Mercury)
eringo
feverfew
figwort
fleabane
foxglove (with Mercury and Saturn)
French mercury
goldenrod
gooseberry
gromwell
ground ivy (with the Sun)
groundsel (common)
herb Robert (with Mars)
herb true-love
hollyhock

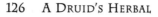

kidneywort
lady's mantle
lentil
lime tree (linden) (with
  Jupiter)
mallow
marshmallow
mayweed (stinking)
mint
moneywort
mother-of-thyme
motherwort
mugwort
orach
orchid
peach tree
pear tree
pennyroyal

pennywort
plantain
ploughman's spikenard
plum tree
primrose
ragwort
raspberry
rocket cress
rose (damask) (with
  Jupiter)
sage (wood)
sanicle
self-heal
silverweed
skirret
soapwort
sorrel (common,
  mountain, sheep's)

sorrel (wood)
sour cherry (morello)
sow thistle (common)
sow thistle tree
spicknel
strawberry (with Sun
  and Jupiter)
sycamore tree
tansy
teasel
thyme (with the Sun)
vervain
violet (with the Moon)
wheat (with Jupiter)
wormwood (with Mars
  and Mercury)
wood sorrel
yarrow

MARS-RULED PLANTS

The herbs of Mars have thorns or prickles and a strong, acrid taste.

Mars is a red-orange planet, and its fiery colors project an aspect as martial as the thorns of its native plants. Mars energy is catalytic and dynamic when used wisely. Used without proper understanding, it degenerates into destructive force.

In the body, Mars rules the muscles, the red blood cells, and the metabolism, including body heat and the transformation of food and oxygen into blood.

Mars rules the motor nerves, the gall, the rectum, the head, the eye muscles, the left half of the brain, and the astral body. Mars also rules the procession of energies from the sexual organs (Scorpio) to the brain pole (Aries)—the kundalini forces.

The left ear, head injuries, inflammations, surgery, the diaphragm, and purgation all fall under the dominion of Mars. Smallpox, scarlet fever, typhus, high blood pressure, fevers, and hemorrhage relate to martial energy, as does intense pain.

Iron, steel, rubies, red corals, and cinnabar are the martial metals and stones. Mars energy, as transmitted by these agents, reaches deep into the animal soul of the human. The instinct for self-preservation is enhanced to a greater degree, and the divine purpose behind that instinct is revealed. Tonics are mixed with herbs of the sun to increase energy, strength, self-reliance, and independence. Spontaneity is evoked in the persona.

Martial herbs can be added to different planetary combinations to enhance the potential of other plants. Passions are stimulated by those plants under the dominion of Mars, and the muscles are toned. Mars energy makes the user passionately gregarious and action-oriented.

Mars enhances the powers of telekinesis. To facilitate the powers of manifestation, combine the herbs of Mars, the Moon, and Mercury.

Some specific herbs of Mars are given here.

For the blood: nettles, all-heal, garlic, hops, cayenne, radish, rhubarb (culinary), sanicle.

For the sex organs: sarsaparilla, garlic, onions, hops, basil.

For the eyes: anemone, crowfoot.

For the muscles: hawthornberry.

HERBS OF MARS

all-heal
aloes (with Saturn)
anemone
arssmart (red shank) (with Saturn)
asarabacca
basil (with Jupiter)
barberry (with Uranus)
blessed thistle
box tree
brooklime
broomrape
bryony
butcher's broom
cacti
capers
capsicum
cardines
catnip

celandine (lesser)
chives
coriander (with Venus)
cotton thistle (down thistle)
crowfoot
cuckoo-pint
daisy (bellis) (with the Moon)
dead nettle
dog rose (with Jupiter)
double rocket (Eve-weed)
dove's foot
down thistle (cotton thistle)
dyer's weed
everlasting flower
Eveweed (double rocket)

flaxweed (with Jupiter and Saturn)
galingale
garlic
gentian (with the Sun and Jupiter)
geranium (herb Robert) (with Venus)
germander
goat's thorn
ground pine
hawthorn tree (with Saturn)
hedge hyssop
honeysuckle
hops
horseradish
horse tongue
leeks
lettuce (wild)

lupine
madder (with Jupiter)
marsh crowfoot (with
  Venus)
masterwort
mezereon (spurge
  laurel)
mustards
nettles
oak tree (with Jupiter)
onions
peppers (cayenne and
  paprika)
pineapple

pine tree
plantain (with the Sun)
radish (black)
rest-harrow
rhubarb (Chinese) (with
  Jupiter)
saltwort
sanicle
sarsaparilla
savine
senna (with Saturn)
shepherd's rod
simson (blue)

sow bread (cyclamen)
stir-thistle
squill
sun spurge
tarragon
tobacco
woodbine (with
  Mercury)
woodruff (squinancy)
woodruff (sweet)
wormseed (treacle)
wormwood (with Venus
  and Mercury)

JUPITER-RULED PLANTS

The plants of Jupiter include edible fruits and nuts as well as plants with a pleasing odor.

Jupiter is the largest planet of our solar system and thus possesses a tremendous magnetic field. When Jupiter and the earth are in conjunction (every 399 days), solar winds carry energies from the magnetic fields of Jupiter to our home planet.

Jupiter rules the liver, the arteries (especially of the abdomen and legs), the fibrin in the blood, subcutaneous fat tissues, adrenalin glands, spleen, kidney, food assimilation, resistance to disease, oxygen in the blood, energy levels, the organs of digestion, thighs, buttocks, sex organs and their blood supply, feet, lungs, ribs, right ear, semen, sugar metabolism, tissue maintenance, and teeth. The pituitary body, with its fluid circulation and growth regulation, fall under Jupiter's sphere.

The diseases of Jupiter stem from immoderate food consumption. Diseases of the blood, lungs, liver, and heart result when Jupiter is badly aspected with other planets. Jovian energy is hyperexpansive and, when poorly aspected, can produce stroke, abscesses, convulsions, and cancer.

In the mineral kingdom, the energies of Jupiter are transmitted by tin, amethyst, lapis lazuli, and blue and yellow sapphires.

The healing plants of Jupiter are those that preserve the body and promote growth. Mentally, they foster an affectionate nature and an intuitive understanding of the cosmic inner meaning of ritual.

Spiritual leaders, healers, lawyers, and those concerned with pomp and circumstance will be benefited in their work. A major feature of Jovian energy is prosperity consciousness, which can attract material as well as spiritual growth and expansion to the individual.

Jupiter herbs bring an appreciation of the great universal laws and the principle of divine grace. Mixed with herbs of the sun, these plant helpers impart an awareness of divine mercy as it applies to evolution.

Jupiter bestows joy and grace. When herbs of Jupiter are mixed with herbs of Mercury, insight will be gained into the philosophical principles of any system and its cosmic significance. This combination puts one in touch with the great avatars, enabling one to learn better and to teach others. The lighthearted gaiety of their combined natures is useful in dispensing depression and gloom.

Some specific herbs of Jupiter are given here.

For the liver: agrimony, balm, costmary, endive, hart's tongue fern, hyssop (hedge), maple leaf and bark, oak, sage, succory (wild), dandelion root.

For the pituitary: wood betony.

HERBS OF JUPITER

agrimony	celandine (with the Sun)	fennel (with Mercury)
alexander	centaury	fig tree (with Venus)
alexandrian parsley	chervil	fir tree
almond (with the Sun)	chestnut tree (with Venus)	flax (with Saturn and Mars)
anise (with Mercury)		
apple tree	chicory (endive) (with Mercury)	fumitory
apricot tree		gentian (yellow) (with the Sun and Mars)
arnica	cinquefoil	
asparagus	clove gilliflower	ginseng
ash tree (with the Sun)	coltsfoot (with Mercury)	goat's beard
avens	comfrey	grapevine (with the Sun)
balm (with the Sun)	costmary	hart's tongue fern
basil	currant	hedge nettle
bay laurel (with the Sun)	dandelion	henbane (with Saturn and Neptune)
beet (white)	docks	
betony (water)	dog's grass	houseleek
betony (wood)	dog rose (with Mars)	hyssop (with Moon and Mars)
blueberry	eglantine	
borage	elecampagne	horse chestnut
carnation	endive (with Mercury)	Irish moss

jessamine
juniper (with the Sun and Mercury)
lady's thistle
lang-de-boeuf
lavender (with the Sun and Mercury)
lemon balm (with Jupiter and the Sun)
licorice (with Mercury)
lichen (dog)
lime tree (linden) (with Venus)
liverwort
lungwort (with Mercury)
madder (with Mars)
manna (flowering ash)
maple tree
marshmallow (with the Sun and Venus)
masterwort
meadowsweet
melilot
mistletoe (with the Sun and Moon)
mullein
mulberry tree
myrrh
nutmeg (with the Moon)
oak tree (with Mars)
oat (with Mercury)
olive (with the Sun)
peppermint (with Venus)
polypody
poplar (with Saturn and the Sun)
raspberry
roses (with Venus)
sage (common garden)
sandalwood (with Venus)
samphire (rock or small)
scarlet pimpernel
scurvy grass
sorrel
succory (wild)
sugar cane
sumac
sycamore tree
swallow-wort
tansy
tomato
thornapple

SATURN-RULED PLANTS

Saturnian plants are cooling in nature. They include woody trees and shrubs that show annual rings, and poisonous or narcotic plants.

Saturn is a cold, dry planet whose character is one of restriction, contraction, and limitation. Saturn is the direct opposite of Jupiter, whose effect it counterbalances. Saturnian forces are a problem only for those who lack self-control. Saturn is a positive influence on the individual who is self-aware and disciplined.

Saturn has been depicted as the ancient guardian of the threshold to the inner mysteries. To the Romans, he was the god of time. All slow and chronic processes are under the influence of Saturn: the aging process, the bones, the teeth (with Jupiter), indurations (hardenings), the anterior lobe of the pituitary (with Jupiter), the spine (with the sun, Neptune, and Leo), the left auricle (when Saturn is in Leo), the endocardium, sterility, bladder, blood composition (with Sun, Jupiter, Venus, and Mars) and circulation to tissues, joints, calves, vertebrae (when Saturn is in Taurus), the assimilation of intestinal fluids, the gall (with Moon, Mercury, Mars), knees, vagus nerve, and spleen (with the Sun and Jupiter).

Diseases of Saturn affect memory and lead to calcification, induration, rheumatism, melancholy, lethargy, lack of sexual desire, and irritable eccentricity.

Lead, onyx, black coral, chalcedony, and lodestone bring the energies of Saturn to the wearer.

Saturn-ruled plants augment the basic structures of life. They impart a sober disposition that will be more prone to accepting the karmic limitations placed upon life. Their quality is steadying, solidifying, subtle, diplomatic, patient, and more suited to work on the physical plane.

These remedies are a grounding force that will enable one to complete projects and realize ideas. Mixed with the essences of Mercury, they enable the student to gain access to, and refine, subtle magical abilities. In general, any herb that is combined with a Saturnian energy will be "earthed," making its work on the physical plane much easier.

Some specific herbs of Saturn are given here.

For the skeleton: comfrey, horsetail, Solomon's seal.

For the cartilage: black poplar, Solomon's seal.

HERBS OF SATURN

aconite (monkshood)
   (with Mars)
amaranthus
aloes (with Mars)
arssmart (redshank)
   (with Mars)
barley
barrenwort
bistort
bearded darnel
   (cockleweed)
beech tree
beets (red)
belladonna (with Mars)
bifoil
birdfoot
bittersweet nightshade
black elder (with Venus
   and Mercury)
blackthorn

blue bottle
buckthorn (alder)
burdock (with Venus)
centaury
chickweed
comfrey (with Jupiter)
clown's woundwort
cornflower
crosswort
cypress
darnel
digitalis (with Mercury
   and Venus)
dodder
elm tree (with Mercury)
eryngo
fenugreek
fern (royal)
flax seed (with Jupiter
   and Mars)

fleawort
fluxweed (flixweed)
fumitory
gall (oak)
goutwort (goutweed)
gladiole (water)
gladwin
hemlock (water)
hawkweed (mouse ear)
   (with the Moon)
hawthorn (with Mars)
hellebore (black)
hemp (with Neptune)
henbane (common)
   (with Jupiter and
   Neptune)
herb Christopher
herb Gerard
holly
horsetail

iris (with the Moon)
Jew's ear
knapweed (common)
knapwort (harshweed)
knotgrass
maize (corn)
male fern
mandrake (with Mercury and Moon)
marijuana
medlar
mezereon spurge
monkshood (aconite) (with Mars)
mullein
nightshade
onion (with Moon and Mars)
pansy
periwinkle (with the Moon)
pine
plantain
polypody root
poplar tree (with Sun and Jupiter)
poppy (with the Moon)
quince tree
root-of-scarcity
royal fern (with the Moon)
rupturewort
rushes
rye
saffron/safflower (meadow) (wild)
sea onion (with Mars)
Scotch pine
sea holly
senna (with Mars)
shepherd's purse
sloe bush (Blackthorn)
Solomon's seal
sorb tree
spleenwort
tamarind
twayblade
violet (water)
water hemlock
wild pansy (heart's ease)
willow herb (hairy)
willow herb (rosebay)
wintergreen
yew tree

CHAPTER 13

Sacred Groves and Circles

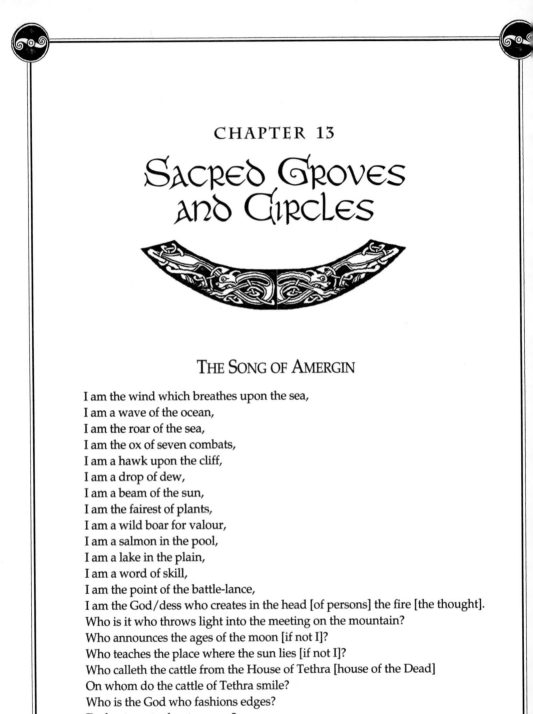

THE SONG OF AMERGIN

I am the wind which breathes upon the sea,
I am a wave of the ocean,
I am the roar of the sea,
I am the ox of seven combats,
I am a hawk upon the cliff,
I am a drop of dew,
I am a beam of the sun,
I am the fairest of plants,
I am a wild boar for valour,
I am a salmon in the pool,
I am a lake in the plain,
I am a word of skill,
I am the point of the battle-lance,
I am the God/dess who creates in the head [of persons] the fire [the thought].
Who is it who throws light into the meeting on the mountain?
Who announces the ages of the moon [if not I]?
Who teaches the place where the sun lies [if not I]?
Who calleth the cattle from the House of Tethra [house of the Dead]
On whom do the cattle of Tethra smile?
Who is the God who fashions edges?
Enchantments about a spear?
Enchantments of wind?

from Dillon, **Early Irish Literature**

Several elements can be considered fundamental to Druidic ritual practice.

Sacred trees, for example, and especially oaks, have played a central role in Druidic rites. The oak is venerated for its great strength and flexibility as well as its practical and healing virtues. A characteristic of the tree is that its roots grow as deep as the tree is high. Thus, it has come to symbolize a balanced life, with head firmly in the celestial spheres and roots solidly in the ground.

Trees have been viewed as vehicles of transformation and rebirth by many cultures. Some examples are the "tree of life," the flowering tree placed at the center of Native American ceremonies; the tree as agent for the shaman's underworld journey (begun by the visualization of an entrance under its roots); the "tree of light" of the Qabbalah; the Judeo-Christian "tree of paradise" at the head of the four rivers (the Edenic tree of knowledge); the Norse cosmic world portrayed as Yggdrasil, the tree from which Odin hung to discover the runes; the Christian "tree" of the cross; and the tree beneath which the Buddha sat to realize enlightenment.

In this context it is easy to understand why Druids perform their most sacred rituals in the presence of an oak.* In choosing sacred sites, hills, stones, trees, wells, and fires have been used as markers to define the mystical center—the place of contact with the Otherworld. The *gorsedd* of Wales and the assemblies of Ireland were traditionally held on hilltops. Celtic and Nordic legends speak of rulers and herdsmen who sat on mounds to issue their commands.

Some meeting places and ritual spaces have been in use for thousands of years. Animal paths may have converged at a certain site, and human hunters soon followed. Eventually, stone pillars or wooden spikes were used to mark the boundaries of these places, which now held the energies of the human and animal traffic.

The stones and spikes were often aligned with solar phenomena such as solstices and equinoxes and with the energies of the Earth's ley lines. Circles are the predominant shape of the sacred enclosures—circles of megaliths, circular groves of trees, and circles of stone that mirror the spheres of the sun and moon and the wheel of the sacred Earth year.

Star lore and moon lore mark the units of time within the ritual year. Festivals are reckoned from dusk to dusk, night being the Goddess's time, best for Otherworldly visits.

---

* The rowan tree held special favor among the Irish Druids, whereas the yew tree was venerated by the British. The oak, while generally revered, was perhaps the most important in Gaul and Galatia.

Spirals, mazes, and the coiled forms of serpents were used by the ancients and are used today as symbols of Earth energies, transformation, and rebirth. Circle dances are performed to energize the Earth. Spiral dances depict the secret process by which the womb of the Mother embraces the seed and sends it forth as a living plant.

Every tree, spring, rock, valley, mountain, and body of water is understood to have its own animating spirit. Each is perceived as a distinct individual with its own store of wisdom to share. Whether conceived of as mirrors reflecting back, more clearly, the impulses and intuitions already held in the psyche, or perceived as spiritual beings in their own right, they reveal the sacred relationship between human, spirit, plant, mineral, and animal: the fundamental infrastructure of the nature religions.

The deities associated with the Druids' groves, of course, are legion, and the reader is urged to study the Mabinogion, the Cycles of Fionn and Arthur, and the Ulster Cycle in order to appreciate their scope.

Rituals are enacted as praise offerings to Gods and Goddesses and as personal and community rites of transformation. Every Druid is expected to develop some bardic skill, and it is in the praise offerings that the power of the bard comes fully into its own. Recitations of poetry, legends, musical compositions, and songs find their fullest expressions in the sacred groves.

Rituals are used as alchemical passages for the individuals and the tribe—opportunities to move from the dark to the light, from the past to the future, and from season to season. The cycles of the ritual year remind us that like the plants that lie fallow in winter to reappear in spring, no psychological or material state persists, and we who *are* life, which is motion, have the continual option of rebirth before us.

Traditional locations for ritual include womb-like entrances to the Earth such as caves. Dolmens—large upright stones covered by a capstone and then covered with earth—may have symbolized earthen caves through which the initiate (or the dead) achieved rebirth. One profound rite of initiation involved the interment of the Druid for three nights and days in a cave or mound. Upon emergence on the third day, she or he was "twice born."

Wells near old oaks or standing stones were especially sacred. Well rituals are still performed today to protect cattle, to keep the fairies in a good humor, and to pray for community and personal needs. A simple rite involves crawling deosil (sunwise) around the well, stone, and tree—three, six, or nine times—after which rags are tied to the tree as personal "prayer flags."

Other common elements of well rituals include drinking the water, bathing parts of the body, using healing stones at the well, dropping pins or small objects into the water, and circumambulating nearby buildings.

At the well of St. Conal, at Inishkeel, Gweebarra Bay, County Donegal, the following ritual is undertaken for the relief of sickness. First, the petitioner removes shoes and stockings, washes the feet carefully, and walks barefoot to a spring. Kneeling to pray at the well, the devotee drinks a little water from a shell and bottles some water to take home. On the grass near the spring are three stone heaps. The petitioner walks three times around each heap, taking stones from the bottom and placing them on top, kneeling after each circumambulation.

The petitioner then proceeds to the east, where a large stone is partially covered with stones left by other pilgrims. One stone is an oval black stone with four parallel white strata on it. The devotee circumambulates the large stone, placing smaller stones on top of it and praying, then takes the oval stone with the white strata, makes the sign of a cross on brow, shoulders, and heart, passes it around the body, and touches it to afflicted parts.

Next comes a climb to the wall of the churchyard and a walk three times around the perimeter of a ruined chapel in the northern section. Prayers are said as the pilgrim walks, bowing while passing the doors on the south side.

After circumambulating the chapel at least three times, the petitioner enters the chapel at the north wall and kneels at the altar, which consists of a stone slab—a fallen dolmen with a round hole at the north end. Four rounded "healing stones" lie on the dolman. The pilgrim kneels before the altar and grinds one of the stones into a round hole, then makes a sign of the cross with each healing stone in turn, passing it round the waist from left to right and applying it to any afflicted body part. Then the pilgrim crosses brow, shoulders, and heart with it again and replaces it on the altar.

Leaving the chapel by the southern doorway, the pilgrim kneels and prays there briefly, perhaps scraping dirt off the doorway and applying it to the afflicted body part, and finally returns to the well and to the previously removed shoes, puts them on, and tears off pieces of rag to place on the rocks near the spring or under or near the altar stone.

Coins are sometimes dropped through the holes in the altar. Rosaries, scapulars, hair pins, and combs are left near by or under the altar.

Tradition holds that water from holy wells cures disease and will drive away rats when sprinkled around the house. The sunwise circumambulations reflect the desire to live in harmony with cosmic forces and the sun, which is seen as the ultimate generator of life.

In Scotland, expectant mothers walk three times sunwise around a church, and wedding parties circumambulate the house three times before entering. Boats are rowed three times in sunwise circles before they set out for fishing. Pots are stirred sunwise, and coffins are carried sunwise around cairns or crosses. These traditions are obviously remnants of pagan sensibilities.

Sacred trees such as hawthorn or hazel are often found near holy wells. The same spirit that inhabits the well is felt to be alive in the tree. The well can be seen as a female energy and the tree as the male principle. Solitary hawthorns growing on hillsides near wells are said to mark the entrance to a fairy mound.

Water has traditionally been seen by Druids as a gateway to the Otherworld. For this reason, deposits are made in springs, wells, and lakes. In Duchcov, Czechoslovakia, two thousand objects—most of them bracelets or brooches—were found in a cauldron in a lake. The Roman consul Caepio found one hundred thousand pounds of gold and one hundred and ten thousand pounds of silver in a Gaulish lake in 106 B.C.E.

Votive deposits in shafts dug in the Earth have included ploughshares, models of swords and shields, pottery, animal and human bones, wooden figures, and even an entire tree trunk. The shafts may be as much as eight feet in diameter and one hundred and twenty feet deep.

As is obvious from the above, the concept of sacrifice and self-sacrifice is intrinsic to the Druid path. Much as when the seed is sacrificed to the earth, and the harvest is sacrificed to the reaper, the Druid sees sacrifice as a way to further the greater life of the community.

Druid initiates begin by sacrificing themselves to learning, to the disciplines of magic, to perfection of their chosen art, and to selfless observance of seasonal rites. The ultimate goal is understood to be spiritual growth for the individual and cultural, spiritual, and material wealth for the clan.

The concept of the ordeal is an ancient one. On a small island off the coast of Ireland, aspirants leave offerings at a holy well at the foot of a hill, climb a narrow trail, squeeze up a chimney-like opening, cross a stone that projects over the sea, and climb to the pinnacle and out on a ledge, four hundred and sixty feet over the ocean, to kiss a stone.

In Locronan, in Brittany, a twelve-kilometer path around a certain hill has twelve stones along its length. Every seven years it is circumambulated by devotees who start in the west and proceed north, east, and south. Then the participants climb the hill and descend by the western slope. On the way down, they walk three times around a large stone representing the moon.

It is well to remember that the ancient Druids often *chose* to be sacrificed for the good of the tribe. It was for this reason that one of Columba's monks asked to be buried alive under a wall at Iona. Many early Irish saints were Druids by birth and training. When they first heard of the sacrifice of Jesus on the tree of the cross, they recognized him as a great Druid and added the sun symbol to the Christian cross. To this day, the Celtic cross is a melding of the solar symbol of the disk and the cross of the Christos.

As scant evidence survives to reveal ancient Druidic liturgical themes, Druids of today are devising original and varied approaches. What follows is an invocation of the directions based loosely on the concepts of Alwyn and Brinley Rees (*Celtic Heritage*, 1961) and of this author's composition.

Powers of the East! From the Fort of Falias, the plain of earth, may we receive Abundance; the cauldron of the Dagda overflowing, milk of the breasts of Boann, spilling over the land and growing to mighty rivers, food, prosperity, beautiful garments, and gainful employ. Come to us now, Salmon of Knowing—teach us to be steadfast and wise. Help us to reap good harvests from fertile soils.

Powers of the South! From the Fort of Murias, fort of the Sea, home of water and of the Night, dark cave of Winter, spirit of Nature and the Land; from the hand of the Goddess may we receive innate knowing, inner vision, and the wisdom of the unconscious. We greet the not-human and the more-than-human; the Little People, the fairies, the pixies, and the elves. Great Stag/Boar* of the South, give us the gifts of Artistry and Craft. Teach us to know the beauty and truth of the stone, the body of the Mother.

Powers of the West! From Findias, shining white fort, may we receive the spears of Enlightenment, Clarity, and Logic. Turn our minds to the love of

---

* Stag in the light half of the year; boar in the dark half.

poetry and of learning. Prepare us to receive the shock of sudden illumination—may it find fertile ground! Wise Boar/Stag,* give us depth and subtlety of intellect. We open to your fire and lightning.

Powers of the North! From Gorias, burning fort of Nuada of the Silver Hand, we receive the sword of Leadership. Teach us to be spiritual warriors, to strive for the good of the community, to be leaders in our nation. Bring to us the blazing white strength of summer's light. Make us perfectly aware, conscious, and awake. Eagle of clear vision, bring to us Courage and Nobility.

Powers of the Center! Sacred tree, Fountain of mead, Fame of queenship and kingship, Place in which and from which all directions meet and flow, we meet thee and greet thee and join thee now! Teach us Balance and Justice and Mastery for all our lives. Great Central Sun, teach us the wisdom of the Sacrifice.[†]

HERBS OF CONSECRATION AND PURIFICATION

Angelica, Asafetida, Basil, Blessed Thistle, Cedar, Elecampane, Frankincense, Fumitory, Hyssop, Juniper, Mandrake, Mistletoe, Oak, Pine, Rosemary, Rowan, Sage, Sandalwood, Tansy, Valerian, Vervain

Please refer to chapter 2, "Herbal Basics," for methods of preparation.

ANGELICA, ANGELICA ARCHANGELICA

Parts Used and Herbal Uses: Please see page 40 in "The Herbs of Imbolc/Oimealg."

Magical Uses: Angelica is burned as incense, placed in the chalice, scattered over the ritual space, and used in the ritual bath.

ARBORVITAE (YELLOW CEDAR), THUJA OCCIDENTALIS

Parts Used and Herbal Uses: Please see page 25 in "The Herbs of Samhain."

---

*Boar in the light half of the year; stag in the dark half.
[†]After the invocation of the center, an oaken staff is symbolically planted in the center of the circle. The circle is now sacred space, beyond the laws of time and matter.

Magical Uses: Cedar smoke purifies the home and ritual space. Use it in smudge sticks, incense, and sweat lodge ceremonies.* The scent is said to enhance psychic powers.

ASAFETIDA, *FERULA FOETIDA*

Part Used: Resin of the root.

Herbal Uses: A plant resin used to treat stomach ailments such as intestinal flu, gas, and bloating. Add a pinch to beans as they cook. The herb is good in cases of *Candida albicans*. Asafetida has been used for asthma, bronchitis, and whooping cough because of its antispasmodic properties and is a good herb for croup and colic in babies (newborns should get it through their mother's milk). Another method is to give it to infants via the rectum—make an emulsion with four parts asafetida to one hundred parts water and insert. It has been used as a sedative for hysteria and convulsions.

PLEASE NOTE: This herb tastes *awful* and is perhaps best taken in capsule form, one hundred milligrams to one gram being the dose.

Magical Uses: Worn in a bag around the neck, asafetida dispels diseases and evils of all kinds. (It literally repels evil spirits!) Add a clove of garlic to enhance the effect. Asafetida is a classic for exorcism and purification rites. Use it to smudge a ritual space with smoke.

BASIL, *OCIMUM BASILICUM*

Parts Used and Herbal Uses: Please see page 41 in "The Herbs of Imbolc/Oimealg."

Magical Uses: Basil brings joy to the user. It creates an aura of understanding between people. Basil is especially appropriate for couples. Use it in incense, in tea, in decorations, and in the ritual bath.

BLESSED THISTLE, *CARDUUS BENEDICTUS = CNICUS BENEDICTUS = CARBENIA BENEDICTA*

Parts Used and Herbal Uses: Please see page 34 in "The Herbs of Meán Geimhridh."

---

*The sweat lodge is a Native American ceremony of purification done outdoors. Young saplings are bent to form a small hut, which is covered with blankets. Hot rocks are brought into the lodge and placed in a hole in the ground, and water is poured over them to produce steam. During the ritual, prayers are said for the Earth, the sky, and the four directions.

Magical Uses: This herb breaks hexes. It protects the wearer from all harm—add it to the chalice and to the ritual bath.

ELECAMPANE (ELFWORT), *INULA HELENIUM*

Parts Used and Herbal Uses: Please see page 188 in "Baby Blessing Herbs."

Magical Uses: Elecampane is burned as incense to bring joy and love. Use it in the ritual chalice.

FRANKINCENSE (OLIBANUM), *BOSWELLIA THURIFERA*, *BOSWELLIA CARTERII*

Parts Used and Herbal Uses: Please see page 35 in "The Herbs of Meán Geimhridh."

Magical Uses: The scent inspires one to reach one's highest spiritual potential. Sacred to the Sun God Ra, frankincense is burned in rites of exorcism, purification, and protection. It is said to accelerate spiritual growth.

FUMITORY, *FUMARIA OFFICINALIS*

Parts Used and Herbal Uses: Please see page 26 in "The Herbs of Samhain."

Magical Uses: Fumitory is burned to exorcise unwanted spiritual entities. Use it in a purification bath preceding your ritual.

HYSSOP, *HYSSOPUS OFFICINALIS*

Part Used: The above-ground portions of the herb.

Herbal Uses: The herb is used (often in combination with sage, which has similar properties, or horehound) for respiratory tract infections. Flu, sore throats, lung complaints, asthma, chronic bronchitis, gas, and bloating are treated by it. Externally, it is used as a wound herb for bruises, injuries, and rheumatism. The green tops of the herb can be added to soups to benefit asthmatics. Hyssop baths are useful for rheumatic complaints. Make a standard infusion of the herb using two teaspoons per cup of water and steeping for twenty minutes. The dose is one-fourth cup four times a day.

Magical Uses: Hyssop was a holy herb of the ancient Greeks, used to cleanse sacred spaces. Hyssop can be burned as incense, worn, used in decorations, and added to the chalice. Use a bunch to ritually "sweep" the altar as a preparation for a ceremonial rite. Alternatively, a tincture can be made (see page 15 for tincture instructions); the dose is ten to thirty drops, four times a day.

JUNIPER, *JUNIPERUS COMMUNIS*

Parts Used and Herbal Uses: Please see page 36 in "The Herbs of Meán Geimhridh."

Magical Uses: Juniper is an herb of protection and purification. It is burned as incense and used to ritually "sweep" an area in preparation for a ritual.

MANDRAKE, *MANDRAGORA OFFICINALIS*

Parts Used and Herbal Uses: Please see page 95 in "Herbs of the Druids."

Magical Uses: Place the root in a vessel of water and expose it to one lunar cycle (new moon to full). Use it to asperge (sprinkle) celebrants and altar.

MISTLETOE, *VISCUM ALBUM*

Parts Used and Herbal Uses: Please see page 100 in "Herbs of the Druids."

Magical Uses: Mistletoe is carried as a protection from all disease and evil influence. It enhances virtually all forms of magical working. Place a few berries in the chalice.

OAK, *QUERCUS* SPP.

Parts Used and Herbal Uses: Please see page 23 in "The Herbs of Samhain."

Magical Uses: Oak is a tree of the sun, sacred to Brighid and the Dagda. Druids do not celebrate unless in the presence of an oak. All parts of the tree are used for magical working as incense, wands, and staves; in ritual baths; and so on. Oak is a tree of healing, abundance, fertility, and strength.

PINE, *PINUS* SPP.

Parts Used and Herbal Uses: Please see page 37 in "The Herbs of Meán Geimhridh."

Magical Uses: Pine is a tree of peace. Burn it to bring joy, purification, and healing. Decorate with its branches for the same effect.

ROSEMARY, *ROSMARINUS OFFICINALIS*

Parts Used and Herbal Uses: Please see page 182 in "House Blessing Herbs."

Magical Uses: Rosemary is an herb of consecration and purification from disease. Add it to incense and to the ritual chalice.

ROWAN, *SORBUS AUCUPARIA*

Parts Used and Herbal Uses: Please see page 62 in "The Herbs of Beltaine."

Magical Uses: Rowan is said to have come from the land of fairy. All parts of the tree are sacred, and it is used for wands, strewn, worn, and burned in incense. Make a tea with a few of the ripe berries and add it to the ritual chalice. Make tiny, equal-armed "solar crosses" as decorations and to be sewn into clothing.

SAGE, *SALVIA OFFICINALIS*

Parts Used and Herbal Uses: Please see page 28 in "The Herbs of Samhain."

Magical Uses: Sage absorbs negativity and misfortune. It drives away disturbances and tensions, and lifts the spirits above the mundane cares of life. Burn it to consecrate a ritual space. Carry it as an herb of protection. Use it in the ritual bath and the chalice.

SANDALWOOD, *SANTALUM ALBUM*

Part Used: Heartwood.

Herbal Uses: The fragrant heartwood is a classic for bladder infections. It is taken to help in the passing of stones, in kidney inflammations, and in prostatitis. The oil is cooling to the body and useful for fevers and infections when used as a massage. The scent is calming to the mind. Sandalwood has been used internally for chronic bronchitis and to treat gonorrhea and the urethral discharge that results. Simmer one teaspoon of the wood per cup of water for twenty minutes, and take up to two cups a day in quarter-cup doses. The alcohol tincture is made according to the directions given on page 15. The dose is twenty to forty drops, four times a day, not with meals.

Homeopathic Uses: Homeopaths use *Santalum* as a remedy for aching in the kidneys.

Magical Uses: Sandalwood oil placed on the forehead aids in focusing the mind. The scent opens the highest spiritual centers and so makes an appropriate incense for rituals, exorcisms, and healings. The powdered wood is strewn to the directions or offered to the fire to bring protection and consecration to any ceremony. Mix it with lavender to enhance contact with the spirit world. Mix it with frankincense for the highest spiritual "octave." The scents of frankincense and sandalwood have some of the highest vibrations inherent in any plant. They will resonate with aspects of ourselves or with Devic/Angelic beings of the highest order. Rose is another herb held to have that frequency, thus attracting or eliciting the highest spiritual vibrations from within ourselves and the cosmos.

TANSY, *TANACETUM VULGARE*

Parts Used and Herbal Uses: Please see page 44 in "The Herbs of Imbolc/Oimealg."

Magical Uses: Tansy is an herb of immortality. Use it in decorations and in the ritual cup.

VALERIAN (ALL-HEAL), *VALERIANA OFFICINALIS*

Part Used: Root.

Herbal Uses: A powerful root for the nerves, valerian should not be taken for longer than a few weeks, as it can become addictive. It helps cure depression when taken once or twice. **CAUTION:** *Valerian produces depression when taken over a long period.* It is a good sedative for such conditions as neuralgia, hypochondria, insomnia, and nervous tension. The tea is strengthening to the eyesight, especially when problems are due to weakness in the optic nerve. Valerian has been used as an anticonvulsant in epilepsy. It slightly slows the heart and thus is a good remedy for palpitations. Simmer two teaspoons of the root in a pint of water for twenty minutes, and take one-fourth cup, cold, four times a day. The tincture can be made according to the directions given on page 15. The dose is twenty drops in water, three times a day. The root is simmered with licorice, raisins, and anise seeds to make a cough sedative. The scent is very attractive to rats and is used to bait traps. Valerian is a warm and spicy herb that has a stimulating effect on the brain as well as being a sedative. If a person has a hot constitution it will be especially stimulating and may negate the calming and sedating quality. A hot constitution is one that is prone to constipation, dryness, redness in the eyes and skin and a warm body temperature (a cold constitution has the opposite qualities).

    CAUTION: *Valerian is best suited to individuals with cold, nervous conditions. Those with heated conditions can experience opposite (i.e., stimulant) effects.*

Homeopathic Uses: Homeopaths use valerian for hysteria, hysterical spasms, hysterical flatulence, hallucinations at night, earache from exposure to cold, sciatica, jerking of the extremities, and long-lasting fevers, and also for children's afflictions, such as the vomiting of curdled milk, diarrhea with lumps of coagulated milk, and much screaming.

Magical Uses: Valerian is added to the chalice as an herb of peace. It is used to asperge the ritual space and in incense for purification. It has been used as a substitute for graveyard dust to repel unwanted presences.

VERVAIN, *VERBENA OFFICINALIS*

Parts Used and Herbal Uses: Please see page 109 in "Herbs of the Druids."

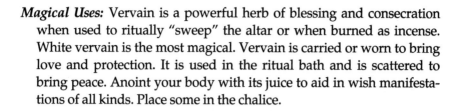

Magical Uses: Vervain is a powerful herb of blessing and consecration when used to ritually "sweep" the altar or when burned as incense. White vervain is the most magical. Vervain is carried or worn to bring love and protection. It is used in the ritual bath and is scattered to bring peace. Anoint your body with its juice to aid in wish manifestations of all kinds. Place some in the chalice.

CHAPTER 14

Last Rites and the Celtic Otherworld

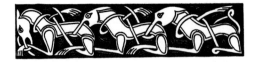

... Lay her in the earth:
And from her fair and unpolluted flesh
May violets spring.

Hamlet, *Act V, scene I*

Those who are wise in spiritual things grieve neither for the dead
nor for the living. I myself never was not, nor thou, nor all the
princes of the earth; nor shall we ever hereafter cease to be. As the
lord of this mortal frame experienceth therein infancy, youth, old
age, so in future incarnations will it meet the same.

Bhagavad Gita

The classical writers testify that the most basic doctrine of the ancient
Druids was the belief in reincarnation. This fundamental religious doctrine was so well accepted that arrangements were sometimes made for
debts to be paid in the Otherworld if left unpaid in this one.

What are the essential characteristics of this Otherworldly realm? It is
located in the West and in the realm of twilight or dawn (intermediate
states between the light half and the dark half of the day). It is a place of
feasting and love, of learning and rest. There is no hellish counterpart.

The Otherworld is essentially a joyful place, described as the "hon-
eyed plain of bliss," the "apple island," the "fortunate island," and the
"summerland."

Druids of today who are recreating and reliving the ancient traditions may choose to journey to the Otherworld in meditation and trance to meet a spiritual guide, to divine a life purpose, to enrich their creative lives, to sensitize themselves to the Earth as a living being, or to meet and interact with the Otherworldly beings who share space with us, often without our knowing it.

To undertake a guided visualization or a poetic journey to the Otherworld, the student must first of all be well grounded, living in a manner characterized by clarity of thought, commitment to spirituality, creativity, practical growth, and integrity. The student should not be in a state where she or he will be swayed by or enamored of any new image or idea that comes along.

No encounter with an Otherworldly being should distract from one's personal sense of spiritual purpose or of rightness or wrongness. Otherworldly etiquette demands humble observation of rules, commonsense precautions, humility, politeness, and a willingness to change but never to compromise one's highest sense of ethics. We, after all, as much as any astral being, are the carriers of divinity in its indwelling, human guise. Our goal is to travel into the Otherworld and return, changed but wiser, and ethically uncompromised, filled with a desire to create our life anew, with a sense that we are fulfilling our personal destiny.

Above all, we need to remember that the Otherworld is a *living* place, one that beckons modern-day voyagers to undertake their own unique adventures to help bring back the shining wisdom that will help us all survive the present dark age of amorality, pollution, and commercial exploitation.

It is beyond the scope of this book to present detailed rituals or processes for journeying. Suffice it to say that traditional means such as shamanic trance drumming, guided visualizations, and vision quests undertaken while fasting are all appropriate methods to gain access to the shining realm.

For Druids, the Otherworld is generally located in areas inaccessible to normal waking vision and hearing. It is sometimes described as under the Earth (in particular, within the Sidhe-mounds, in the realm of fairy), or under the waves. It is often said to be on an island or a series of islands, on the other side of a mist, on an open plain, or beyond the horizon.

It is a place of battles undertaken for the sheer exuberance of spirit, and feasting, and peace; a place of radiantly divine women and hags; a place of hunters, heroes, and craftsmen; a place of goodness and monstrous evil, beyond time as the "middle world" understands it.

It is the place of the union of opposites and irreconcilables, which can only be reached by a bridge as thin as a razor's edge—a place beyond space, the perfect, never-quite-realized center of things, characterized in our world by the spaces between day and night or between the dark half and the light half of the year. Much like the sacred mistletoe—neither shrub nor tree, living above and below, yet belonging to neither sphere entirely—it is free from the limitations of intellectual classification. Breaking the bonds of the rational, existing between the realm of chaos and the ultimate ground of all being, it is the enigma that splits pure reason to reveal the subconscious architecture of the universal mind.

Of course, the final and most profound Otherworldly journey takes place after the dissolution of the physical body. At this time, the relation of the body to earthly life is shattered by burning or by disintegration into the soil and air. Chants are sung and verses recited that will help the deceased in the transition from this world to the next.

Boat burials have traditionally been performed by casting the body to sea in a vessel, or by placing a boat in the tomb. A tree such as an oak is sometimes hollowed out to admit the body on its final voyage.

Weapons, chariots (a car might be the modern Druid's equivalent offering), provisions for feasting (including wine and enough fare for guests), and hunting gear can be placed in the grave. Jewelry and robes are lovingly added by friends and kin. Personal items are smashed and added as a token that they are meant for Otherworldly use.

After a funeral, the family and friends visit the grave from time to time to tell the deceased about family events. Dishes of food are left at Samhain as a gift for the spirit of the departed.

In *The Voyage of Maeldúin*, thirty-three islands are described. These wondrous stations are possibly a recounting of the soul's progress through various after-death states, serving a function similar to the *Bardo Thödol, The Tibetan Book of the Dead*, which is read by a priest (lama) at the time of death to edify the deceased as well as the grieving family.

The deity invoked at death rites is Mannanán Mac Lir, god of the headlands, Son of the Sea, patron of death, rebirth, ancestors, and sailors. Possessor of "the crane bag" of power, he rides a magical horse who carries voyagers to the Otherworld across the seas. Mannanán may appear as a warrior on a dark gray steed with a golden bridle, who submerges and reappears in the ocean swells, yet never gets wet.

In common with the Greek tradition of dolphins who carry souls under and above the waves by turns until they arrive, reborn, in the islands of the blessed, Mannanán can be seen to symbolize a consciousness that can navigate the inner and outer worlds with impunity until it reaches the Otherworld kingdom of Tír Tairngire.

HERBS FOR FUNERALS

Aconite, Asphodel, Basil, Bean, Bluebell, Chervil,
Elder, Hawthorn, Lotus, Mandrake, Marjoram, Myrrh, Parsley,
Pasque Flower, Pennyroyal, Periwinkle, Pine, Poplar, Rosemary,
Rue, Star Anise, Tansy, Thyme, Violet, Willow, Yew

Please refer to chapter 2, "Herbal Basics," for methods of preparation.

ACONITE (MONKSHOOD, WOLFBANE), *ACONITUM NAPELLUS*

Part Used: Root.

> **CAUTION:** *This plant is poisonous and must be used with professional supervision.* A small amount taken internally can cause death, and its juice was once applied to arrow tips to kill wolves. The roots are dug in autumn and dried.

Herbal Uses: Aconite has been added to salves because of its painkilling action on neuralgia, lumbago, and rheumatism. The tincture has been given in *one-drop doses* for heart failure, high fevers, pneumonia, pleurisy and tonsillitis. Because of its *deadly nature*, herbal aconite should probably be avoided.

Homeopathic Uses: Homeopathic aconite, however, is another story, being *very* dilute and completely safe. Homeopaths use *Aconitum napellus* for conditions of mental and physical restlessness; fear and shock; a great fear of death; acute, sudden, and violent fevers; conditions brought on by dry, cold weather and winds; and influenza. Vinegar given in large amounts can antidote its effects.

Magical Uses: Aconite brings protection from werewolves and vampires.

Aconite was a classic component of flying ointments, which generally also contained henbane, belladonna, hemlock, and soot. Without the blessings of the angel of death, no new life would be possible, and so we honor death and the dead by burning aconite as funeral incense and by planting it on a loved one's grave.

ASPHODEL, ASPHODELUS RAMOSUS

Part Used: Root.

Herbal Uses: A Mediterranean root, asphodel is taken to promote menstruation and is used as an antispasmodic. Simmer two teaspoons per cup and take one-fourth cup four times a day. The poultice of asphodel is applied externally to swellings and infections. Please see page 15 for directions on how to make a poultice.

Magical Uses: In ancient times, the white asphodel was planted on graves, as it was considered to be a favorite food of the dead. (Asphodel can be roasted in ashes and eaten, or dried and boiled and added to bread dough.) One could leave an offering of the cooked root or bread on a grave as a gift for the departed. This herb is also used to ritually bathe a corpse.

BASIL, OCIMUM BASILICUM

Parts Used and Herbal Uses: Please see page 41 in "The Herbs of Imbolc/Oimealg."

Magical Uses: Basil is burned as incense, strewn onto floors, and used in purification baths. An open bowl of basil placed in a room dispels melancholy.

BEANS, PHASEOLUS SPP.

Beans were distributed and eaten at funerals in ancient Rome and are still given out to the poor in Italy on the anniversary of a death. Beans are associated with the underworld. Dry beans, though apparently lifeless, carry within them a visibly complete plant embryo and the potential to manifest new life.

BLUEBELLS, *Hyacinthus nonscriptus, Scilla nutans*

Part Used: Dried, powdered bulb.

A wild, perennial bulb, bluebell must be dried before use.

Herbal Uses: Dried and powdered, a dose of three grains (195 milligrams) is given for leucorrhoea. It is also diuretic and styptic.

CAUTION: *An overdose will cause poisoning, as will the use of the fresh bulb. This herb is not recommended for domestic use.*

Magical Uses: This flower is known as the "hyacinth of the ancients," a flower associated with mourning and grief. Apollo and Zephyr both loved the youth Hyacinth; but Hyacinth preferred Apollo. Seeking revenge, Zephyr broke up a game of quoits that Hyacinth was playing by blowing a quoit at Hyacinth, who was killed by it. In his grief, Apollo created the hyacinth flower out of the youth Hyacinth's blood. This herb is planted on graves as a token of grief and used to decorate the altar.

CHERVIL, *Myrrhis odorata*

Parts Used: Above-ground portion of the herb, and root.

Herbal Uses: The juice of the flowering herb is taken internally for skin conditions such as eczema and scrofula. The fresh or dry herb is taken as tea for gout, abscesses, or edema; to bring on menstruation; for anemia; and to lower blood pressure. The fresh root can be eaten, used in decoction, or tinctured. Follow the standard method for decoction: two teaspoons of herb per cup, simmered for twenty minutes and taken in quarter-cup doses, four times a day; or a tincture can be made according to the directions on page 15. The dose is ten to twenty drops, four times a day. Use the roots externally as an antiseptic wound wash or internally for coughs, gas, and upset stomach. Chervil is used in salves for ulcers, wounds, and gout. Follow the general directions for salves given on page 14. The plant can be used safely over a long period of time and is quite harmless; it can be given freely.

CAUTION: *Chervil resembles hemlock (Conium maculatum), which is a deadly poison and must be identified with care.*

Magical Uses: Chervil is added to the ritual chalice or burned in incense to aid in communion with the spirit of the departed. Chervil, an herb of immortality, helps us to commune with our own eternal nature, which transcends the body, space, and time.

ELDER, *SAMBUCUS NIGRA*

Parts Used and Herbal Uses: Please see page 69 in "The Herbs of Meán Samhraidh."

Magical Uses: Elder is a sacred wood used in funeral pyres. Sprigs of elder—a Goddess tree—are placed in the coffin.

HAWTHORN, *CRATAEGUS* SPP.

Parts Used and Herbal Uses: Please see page 59 in "The Herbs of Beltaine."

Magical Uses: Hawthorn was a ritual tree of the ancient Teutons. Sacred to Thor, its wood was used to build funeral pyres. It was believed that the souls of the dead would escape via the burning thorns, and so ascend to the heavens.

LOTUS, *NELUMBO NUCIFERA*

Parts Used: Leaf, node of the root, buds, and seeds.

Herbal Uses: The leaf of *Nelumbo nucifera* is used for fever, sweating, irritability, dysentery, diarrhea, and scanty urine. It is a styptic (stops bleeding) and has been used to antidote alcohol and mushroom poisoning. It affects liver, heart, and spleen energies. The nodes of the root are used to stop bleeding and to break down blood clots. All types of internal bleeding are affected. The plumule (bud) affects the heart, kidney, and spleen. It is used to calm mental agitation and worry, relieve insomnia, and lower fevers. The seed affects the kidney, heart, and spleen. It is used for agitation, insomnia, palpitations, dry mouth, dark urine, and chronic diarrhea. It strengthens the heart and kidneys.

The leaf is steeped, and the bud, root, and seed are simmered, using two teaspoons of herb per cup of water, for twenty minutes. The dose is one-fourth cup, four times a day.

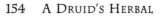

Magical Uses: Lotus is an all-purpose spiritual elixir. Burned as incense, it encourages the dead to seek their highest possible reincarnation. It reminds the living of their inner sanctity and divinity. Lotus plants thrive in murky waters. They float serenely on the stagnant surface and never a drop sticks to them.

MANDRAKE, *MANDRAGORA OFFICINALIS*

Parts Used and Herbal and Magical Uses: Please see page 95 in "The Herbs of the Druids."

MARJORAM, *ORIGANUM MAJORANA*; WILD MARJORAM, *O. VULGARE*

Part Used: Above-ground portions of the herb.

Herbal Uses: The oil of marjoram is useful in killing pain. A drop can be placed on an aching tooth. Marjoram tea promotes perspiration and brings eruptive conditions such as measles to a head. The warm tea is helpful for spasms, colic, and upset stomach. A fomentation of the herb tea is used for swollen joints and rheumatism. A tea of the fresh herb relieves headaches. The tea has been used to bring on menstruation, and in baths and inhalations to clear bronchi and lungs. Make a standard infusion using two teaspoons of the herb per cup of water. The dose is one-quarter cup, four times a day.

Homeopathic Uses: Homeopaths use *Origanum* for nervous conditions and excessive sexual impulses, especially when there is an obsessive desire for exercise and running.

Magical Uses: Marjoram was an herb of happiness to the ancient Greeks, who placed it on graves to bring joy to the deceased. It was also used in bridal wreaths. Use it to bring someone out of a depression.

MYRRH, *COMMIPHORA MYRRHA*

Parts Used and Herbal Uses: Please see page 44 in "The Herbs of Imbolc/Oimealg."

Magical Uses: Myrrh was at one time used by the ancient Egyptians in embalming mixtures and as incense.

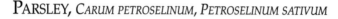

PARSLEY, *CARUM PETROSELINUM, PETROSELINUM SATIVUM*

Parts Used: Root, leaf, and seed.

Herbal Uses: The second-year roots, the leaf, and the seed are used. Parsley is diuretic and helpful for gravel and stone as well as for edema, jaundice, and kidney problems. The root is the most powerful part. The oil of the seed (five to fifteen drops) has been used to bring on menstruation. The seed, when decocted, has been used for intermittent fevers. Steep one teaspoon of leaf per cup for twenty minutes or simmer one teaspoon of the root or seed for twenty minutes. The dose is one-fourth cup, four times a day. Parsley leaves (with violet leaf and figwort herb when possible) are used in poultices for cancer. Follow the standard directions for poultices given on page 15. A parsley poultice will help insect bites, stings, and sore eyes. Parsley tea is used for asthma and coughs.

CAUTION: *Persons with weak kidneys should avoid this herb.*

Homeopathic Uses: Homeopaths use *Petroselinum* for very itchy hemorrhoids, as well as for urinary complaints such as a deep itch in the urinary tract, and gonorrhea with a sudden urge to urinate and a milky discharge.

Magical Uses: Parsley was used in funeral rites by the Greeks; it was held sacred to Persephone. It was wound into funeral wreaths and used to decorate tombs.

PASQUE FLOWER (PULSATILLA), *ANEMONE PULSATILLA*

Parts Used: Above-ground portions of the herb, and root.

Herbal Uses: The tincture of the flowering plant is used for digestive disturbances and illness involving the mucous membranes of the lung. Coughs, asthma, bronchitis, and whooping cough have been treated with pulsatilla. Mucous conditions in the eye and in diarrhea are addressed by it. Headaches, neuralgia, suppressed menstruation, and nervous exhaustion fall under its sphere. The tincture is made from the fresh plant, following the directions on page 15. The dose is two to three drops in water, four times a day. Chinese herbalists use the root for amebic and bacterial dysentery and as a douche for vaginal trichomonas. Follow the standard method for decoction: use two teaspoons per cup and simmer for twenty minutes. Take one-fourth cup, four times a day. Because of its delicate composition, the tincture will last only about a year.

   CAUTION: *Overdose or overuse can cause depression, upset stomach, and nervousness. Pasque flower can be fatal if taken in large amounts.*

Homeopathic Uses: Homeopaths use *Pulsatilla* for conditions of changeable or contradictory nature. All symptoms are better when the person is in open air and undergoing gentle motion, even when the person is chilly and ill. Sadness and weeping are characteristics calling for this remedy, as are thick, bland, yellowish-green discharges. Fat foods, warm foods, and hot liquids make the patient worse. They will be better while receiving cold foods and applications, and worse in the evening hours.

Magical Uses: The anemone flower tends to droop gracefully and, in Greek legend, is said to have grown from the tears that Venus shed as she wept for the dead Adonis. For this reason, it is planted on graves.

PENNYROYAL, *MENTHA PULEGIUM, HEDEOMA PULEGIOIDES*

Part Used: Above-ground portions of the herb.

Herbal Uses: Pennyroyal tea is a classic remedy for menstrual problems and for colds. Use two teaspoons of herb per cup of water, steep for twenty minutes, and take one-fourth cup four times a day. The tea is safe for children in small, frequent doses.

   The oil of pennyroyal can be rubbed directly on the abdomen to relieve menstrual cramps. It is also an effective natural mosquito repellent; mix it with citronella to repel flying and biting insects.

   In ancient times, pennyroyal was hung in the sickroom and in sleeping quarters. Pennyroyal tinctured in vinegar is used as a wash for ulcers, burns, bruises, and even leprosy. Spasms, hysteria, gas, and stomach upset are helped by it. Follow the standard instructions for tincturing as given on page 15, but *do not use alcohol.* You should use good apple cider vinegar instead.

   CAUTION: *This herb can be abortive and should be avoided during pregnancy.* CAUTION: *Do not ingest the oil.*

Homeopathic Uses: Homeopaths use *Mentha pulegium* for pain in the bones of the forehead and extremities.

Magical Uses: Pennyroyal is an herb of protection when worn or carried. Tied on the bed post, it sharpens the brain and wits. Penny-royal kept in a bowl brings peace to the household. It is used to bathe the body of the deceased to bring about a peaceful transition to the next life.

PERIWINKLE, *VINCA MINOR, V. MAJOR*

Parts Used: Above-ground portions of the herb, and flowers.

Herbal Uses: The herb is a familiar woodland groundcover, which bears blue flowers in spring. It is brewed as a tea for diarrhea, heavy menstruation, and hemorrhages. Chewing the plant relieves toothache. The tea is sedative and is beneficial for hysteria, fits, and nervous states. Use two teaspoons per cup, steep for twenty minutes, and take in quarter-cup doses four times a day. Make a poultice of the herb to relieve cramps in the limbs. The leaves are used in salves for hemorrhoids and inflammations. Follow the standard directions for salves and poultices on pages 14 and 15. Use the tea as a gargle for sore throat and tonsillitis. The fresh flowers are made into a syrup laxative, which is excellent for small children as well as adults. To make a syrup, boil three pounds of Sucanat (dessicated sugar cane juice) in one pint of water until you get a syrup consistency, and then steep the herbs in the hot liquid for twenty minutes, or simmer the herbs in honey or maple syrup for about ten minutes, strain, and store in the refrigerator (use two teaspoons of the herb per cup of liquid).

Homeopathic Uses: Homeopaths use *Vinca minor* in low potencies as a remedy for oozing eczema, mild itching, hemorrhages, and diphtheria.

Magical Uses: Once called "sorcerer's violet," periwinkle is used in love charms and potions. A powerful charm against evil spirits, it was also called the "flower of death," as it was made into crowns for dead children at their burial. In Germany it was known as the "flower of immortality," and in France it symbolized friendship. One should never bring fewer than seven blossoms into the house.

PINE, *PINUS SPP.*

Parts Used and Herbal Uses: Please see page 37 in "The Herbs of Meán Geimhridh."

Magical Uses: Pine is evergreen and is an herb of immortality. Its wood is used to make coffins, and its boughs are placed on graves to remind the living that life is eternal and death but a transition to a different reality. Burn the needles to bring harmony and healing to the bereaved.

POPLAR, *POPULUS BALSAMIFERA, P. NIGRA, P. TREMULOIDES, P. CANDICANS, P. GRANDIDENTATA*

Parts Used: Bark and buds.

Herbal Uses: The bark of *P. tremuloides* is used in decoctions for fevers, urinary infection, and gonorrhea. The sticky, resinous winter buds of all poplars are used internally as tea, and externally in salves for coughs, sore throats, cuts, scratches, wounds, and burns. The buds of *P. nigra* (black poplar) are made into a tea to help arthritis and rheumatism. To prepare the bark or bud as tea, simmer two teaspoons of plant per cup of water for twenty minutes, strain, and take one-fourth cup four times a day. To make the salve follow the guidelines for salves given on page 14.

Homeopathic Uses: Homeopaths use *P. candicans* (balm of Gilead) in tincture for acute colds with loss of voice. *P. tremuloides* (American aspen) is used for bladder problems, night sweats, indigestion, nausea, and enlarged prostate.

Magical Uses: In ancient Greece, the black poplar was a funeral tree, held sacred to the Earth Mother. In ancient Ireland, the *fe,* or measuring rod used by coffin makers, was made of poplar wood. In Mesopotamia, corpses were decorated with golden headdresses of poplar. Its trembling leaves are said to be sensitive to the messages of the Gods, Goddesses, and spirits, which drift in the winds.

ROSEMARY, *ROSEMARINUS OFFICINALIS*

Parts Used and Herbal Uses: Please see page 182 in "House Blessing Herbs."

Magical Uses: Rosemary is carried in the hand during funerals and is cast onto the coffin as it is lowered into the grave.

RUE, *Ruta graveolens*

Part Used: Above-ground portions of the herb.

Herbal Uses: CAUTION: *Some people may experience skin irritation when picking the fresh plant.* The whole herb is used, fresh or dry. It is taken warm to bring on menstruation. The infusion benefits coughs, cramp, and colic. Steep two teaspoons of the dried herb in a cup of water for twenty minutes. Take no more than one-half cup per day. The leaves are used in poultices and salves to relieve sciatica, gout, and rheumatic pains. Follow the standard directions for poultices and salves on pages 14 and 15. The fresh leaves are placed on the temples to relieve headache. Fomentations of the tea are placed on the chest to help bronchitis. The juice or oil is placed in the ear to relieve earaches. Eaten in salads (a leaf or two only!), it clears the eyesight.

The fresh juice can be mixed with honey as a preservative and applied to the eyes (one drop, two or three times a day) to sharpen vision and relieve overstrained eyes. Mixed with hot water, the honey-rue combination can be used as a gargle or a tea for colds, flu, and stomach disorders. Use only one teaspoon of the fresh juice over the period of one day.

CAUTION: *This is a strong herb. Use in dosages only as indicated. Overdose will lead to vomiting.*

Homeopathic Uses: Homeopaths use *Ruta graveolens* for eyestrain, strained tendons, sprains (after arnica has been used), bruised bones, constipation, colon cancer, pain in the thighs upon stretching, and headache that follows eyestrain. All symptoms are worse when the patient is lying down or in cold, wet weather. The tincture diluted with ten parts water can be used as a lotion for the eyes.

Magical Uses: A powerful herb of purification. Rue water is sprinkled around a ritual site, or a branch of rue is used to sprinkle salt water. Rue brings protection and clears negativity.

STAR ANISE, *Illicium anisatum, I. verum*

Part Used: Seed.

Herbal Uses: Chew the seeds after a meal to help the digestion. Simmer the seeds to make a tea for colic and rheumatic complaints. Steep one teaspoon of the crushed seed in one cup of boiled water for twenty minutes, and take up to two cups a day. Often added to other brews to improve taste, the tea of the seed will help cramps and nausea, promote menstruation, and increase breast milk. It also relieves insomnia. The seeds are simmered into salves for scabies and lice. Follow the standard directions for salves on page 14. The oil is a stomach tonic. The seeds can be tinctured in brandy with some lemon peel; the dose is one-fourth to one-half teaspoon. Use the method described under tincture preparation on page 15. Use brandy instead of the usual vodka, whiskey, or grain alcohol.

Homeopathic Uses: Homeopaths use *Illicium* for long-standing colic with a pain in the region of the third rib, as well as for asthma, epilepsy, and cough with pus-like phlegm.

Magical Uses: The powdered bark is used in incense. The tree is planted by the Japanese around temples and on graves as an herb of consecration and protection.

TANSY, *TANACETUM VULGARE*

Parts Used and Herbal Uses: Please see page 44 in "The Herbs of Imbolc/Oimealg."

Magical Uses: Tansy was once used in embalming preparations. A branch of tansy is an appropriate herb to use in asperging a body, a gravesite, or a ritual area.

THYME, *THYMUS VULGARIS*

Part Used: Above-ground portions of the herb.

Herbal Uses: Thyme is an excellent lung cleanser. Use it to dry up and clear out moist phlegm and to treat whooping cough. It makes a good tea for the mother after childbirth, as it helps expel the placenta. Steep one-half teaspoon fresh herb or one teaspoon dried herb in one-half cup of hot water for five minutes. Take up to one and a half cups a day in quarter-cup doses. A natural antiseptic, thyme is often used in salves for wounds, swellings, sciatica, and failing eyes. Follow the standard instructions for salves given on page 14. The tea relieves gas and colic (as does the oil, taken in one- to five-drop doses). The tincture can be used in ten- to twenty-drop doses, taken three times a day (follow the standard instructions for tincture given on page 15). Use thyme for headaches and hangovers.

Homeopathic Uses: Homeopaths use *Thymus serpyllum* (wild thyme) in tincture for children's respiratory infections, nervous asthma, and whooping cough, especially when accompanied by ringing in the ears and a burning sore throat.

Magical Uses: Thyme is burned in incense to purify an area. It is worn or added to the ritual cup to aid in communing with the deceased. (It also helps one to see Otherworldly entities such as fairies.) A place where wild thyme grows will be a particularly powerful energy center on the Earth.

VIOLETS, *VIOLA ODORATA*

Parts Used and Herbal Uses: Please see page 45 in "The Herbs of Imbolc/Oimealg."

Magical Uses: Violets and periwinkle are used to decorate the graves and corpses of children.

WILLOW, *SALIX NIGRA, SALIX ALBA*

Part Used: Bark, collected in the spring.

Herbal Uses: Black willow (*S. nigra*) bark is used to treat gonorrhea and ovarian pain. The white willow (*S. alba*) contains salicin, the active constituent from which aspirin was first synthesized. White willow bark is used for rheumatic complaints, arthritis, and headaches as well as diarrhea and dysentery. Fevers, edema, and the aftereffects of worms are treated with willow bark. To make the tea, steep three teaspoons of the bark in one cup of cold water for two to five hours, boil for one minute, and strain. Willow is also available as a powder. The dose is one teaspoon, three times a day in tea or capsules. The tincture can be taken in ten- to twenty-drop doses four times a day.

Homeopathic Uses: Homeopaths use *Salix nigra* for gonorrhea, ovarian pain, bleeding uterine fibroids, painful testicles, blocked menstruation, and back pain. The remedy is also useful in mental conditions: hysteria, nervousness, and excessive sexual passion.

Magical Uses: Willows are commonly found near ancient British burial sites. The willow is a guardian tree, said to protect from evil influences. The willow tree has a healing aura that blesses all it touches.

YEW, *TAXUS BACCATA*

Parts Used: Needles, tips of branches, bark, and berry.

Herbal Uses: Do not use this plant without professional supervision. The only harmless part is the red fleshy portion of the berry. However, the needles and branch tips have been used for lung and bladder problems, arthritis, gout, and pustular skin diseases under strict professional supervision (yew is a violent purgative). Recently a new cancer drug, Taxol, has been derived from its bark and needles.

    CAUTION: *This plant is poisonous.*

Homeopathic Uses: Homeopaths prepare an alcohol tincture of *Taxus baccata* for the conditions just described, especially when accompanied by bad-smelling night sweats. The homeopathic solution is dilute and completely safe.

Magical Uses: This plant is burned to contact the spirits of the dead. Because it grows to a great age, it became a symbol of stability in Celtic regions. It was used as the central "world tree" in ritual spaces and was often planted in graveyards.

    Yew sends up new trees from its roots, so it is a powerful symbol of death and reincarnation. Yew wood is appropriate for magical tools such as wands and staves. In ancient times yew sticks were carved with the Ogham characters as tools of divination.

CHAPTER 15

Under the Marriage Oak

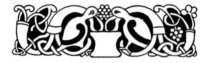

Come live with me and be my love,
And we will all the pleasures prove
That valleys, groves, hills and fields,
Woods or steepy mountains yield.

And we will sit upon the rocks
Seeing the shepherds feed their flocks
By shallow rivers, to whose falls
Melodious birds sing madrigals.

And I will make thee beds of roses
And a thousand fragrant posies,
A cap of flowers, and a kirtle
Embroidered all with leaves of myrtle;

A gown made of the finest wool,
Which from our pretty lambs we pull;
Fair linéd slippers for the cold,
With buckles of the purest gold;

A belt of straw and ivy buds,
With coral clasps and amber studs;
And if these pleasures may thee move,
Come live with me and be my love.

The shepherd swains shall dance and sing
For thy delight each May morning;
If these delights thy mind may move,
Then live with me and be my love.

Christopher Marlowe,
"The Passionate Shepherd to His Love"

To divine whether you will marry your lover, drop two acorns into a pan of water. If the nuts come together, a match is certain. When you have made your choice, remember that Beltaine is the proper time for wooing and that marriage is best when undertaken at Lugnasad or in the dark half of the sacred year.

Marriage is a profound commitment, not to be undertaken lightly. The ancient Celtic Brehon laws recognized nine types of marriage, only one of which was permanent. One common Celtic marriage contract was for a year and a day. Only one arrangement was expected to last indefinitely, yet even then both parties had the right to divorce.

The "permanent" marriage involved an economic exchange—both families gave goods or money and in the event of a divorce the parents of the bride and groom kept their portions. Grounds for divorce included cruelty and adultery. If a man desired a second wife or a concubine, he had to have his first wife's permission.

A divorced woman took her property with her when she returned to her parents' tribe. A married woman remained a member of the tribe of her birth—even though she might move in with the clan of her husband.

Property was passed down through the father's line, though the ancient Picts were apparently matrilineal. In all types of marriage, whichever partner had the most wealth was the partner in control. Upper class women with their own wealth had lovers as they pleased.

Another type of marriage was one where the couple eloped. No dowries were exchanged and so it was understood that they belonged to and had obligation to no tribe or clan—they were people without property living on their own.

An interesting type of marriage was one, fully sanctioned by the law, involving two lunatics, in which it was understood that they would have sexual relations yet be exempt from obligations to either clan.*

---

* For more on this see Jean Markale, *Women of the Celts*, Inner Traditions International, Rochester, Vt., 1986.

Traditional weddings and handfastings (the Pagan ceremony) are often performed under the marriage oak. Pagan partners have the option of choosing the length of their union. It can be for "a year and a day," or for thirteen years, or for a lifetime. The couple makes the decision. The newly joined couple then dances under the tree. In the Orkneys, engaged couples clasp hands through a hole in the Stone of Odin to pledge themselves to each other. At Kirk Braddan on the Isle of Man, the same ritual gesture is used as part of the wedding ceremony.

Weddings can be held inside stone circles within which the participants dance. Newly married couples might circumambulate a stone while asking for fertility, or pass naked through a large hole carved out of a stone (symbolic of rebirth into their new life).

The bride is the earthly representative of spiritual treasure, which must be fought for with determination and courage. She symbolizes the Otherworld and a previously unexplored region of the groom's psyche. The groom embodies the assertive male energy that must accomplish worldly deeds. Spiritually and physically, the couple must overcome the obstacles to their union in order for each to become whole.

For these reasons, displays of mock hostility, the blocking of entrances and gates, and the creation of rope barriers to test the couple's determination are part of the rite. Hostile spirits are dispelled by loud noises. Mock insults and weapons may be used against the bride's party, and the bride may even be placed on a horse to be pursued by her dismayed kin, who must attempt to get her back. Conversely, a relative of the bride might carry her off, with the groom and his party in hot pursuit.

When everyone tires of the game, the groom is "allowed" to claim the bride, and the celebrations and feasting begin.

An alternative to the horseplay might be to challenge the groom to solve a riddle. Or the bride's people and the groom's people can challenge each other to a contest in verse.

An old Welsh custom is for the bride to disguise herself; one of the groom's men is supposed to pick her out of the gathered crowd.

After the ceremony, an old woman meets the bride and presents her with a bag of hazelnuts—symbolic of the wisdom and the creativity she will enjoy in her new life's passage.

HANDFASTING HERBS

Anise, Apple, Broom, Caraway, Coriander, Damiana,
Elderflower, Ginger, Holly, Ivy, Jasmine, Lavender, Lemon Verbena,
Licorice, Lotus, Maple, Marjoram, Meadowsweet, Mistletoe,
Orchid root, Quince, Rose, Rosemary, Skullcap, Yarrow

Please refer to chapter 2, "Herbal Basics," for methods of preparation.

ANISE, *PIMPINELLA ANISUM*

Part Used: Seed.

Herbal Uses: The seeds are carminative (they move gas out of the in-testinal tract). Used in tea or as lozenges, they soothe a hard cough. For the tea, steep one teaspoon of the seeds in one cup of boiled water for ten minutes. Take up to one and a half cups a day. The seeds can also be tinctured using two ounces of seed per one-half quart of brandy and some lemon peel. Let the mixture sit for twenty days. The dose is one teaspoon as needed. The seeds are made into a liquor called anisette, which is mixed with hot water as a remedy for bron-chitis and asthma. Anise seed tea is sweetened with honey and given to children with lung colds. Epilepsy, colic, and smoker's cough are treated with anise. For colic, simmer one teaspoon of the seed in one-half pint of milk for ten minutes, strain, and take it hot. Oil of anise is a natural insecticide.

Magical Uses: Anise seeds are an herb of protection, said to avert all evil. In ancient Roman times, they were baked into a cake that was served at the end of the wedding feast.

APPLE, *MALUS* SPP.

Parts Used and Herbal Uses: Please see page 24 in "The Herbs of Sam-hain."

Magical Uses: Apples and apple blossoms are symbolic of love, heal-ing, and immortality. Burn the blossoms as incense, wear the per-fume, and make them into herb candles for the rite.

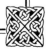

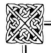

BROOM, *Cytisus scoparius*

Parts Used: Flowering twig and seed.

Herbal Uses: Flowering broom tips are gathered in spring (before Mid-summer) and are later used fresh or dry. The seeds are as useful as the tops. Both are soluble in water and alcohol. The infusion is used to treat cardiac edema. Simmer one teaspoon of the herb or seeds per cup of water for twenty minutes. The dose is one-half cup a day in one-fourth cup doses. Broom is combined with dandelion root, uva ursi, and juniper berries to treat bladder and kidney ailments. Take one part broom, one half part uva ursi, and one half part dandelion root. Simmer until the liquid is reduced to half the original quantity. Add one-half part juniper berry and cool. A pinch of cayenne is sprinkled into each one-eighth cup dose. CAUTION: *Acute kidney problems contraindicate this herb.* Broom is a heart tonic. Use one teaspoon of the herb per cup of water, and *do not exceed more than one-half cup per day.* One to ten drops of tincture may be given as a dose. Follow the standard directions for tinctures given on page 15.

CAUTION: *Overdose can severely weaken the heart or even result in death.*

Homeopathic Uses: Homeopaths use *Cytisus scoparius (Spartium scoparium)* to reduce blood pressure and for edema and kidney infections. It helps the heart after morphine withdrawal and angina pectoris.

Magical Uses: Broom flowers bound with colored ribbons are carried at weddings. Couples may choose to "jump the broom" as they make their transition to a new station in life. Use broom to ritually sweep a space for a magical working. Toss it in the air or bury it to raise or calm winds.

CARAWAY, *Carum carvi*

Part Used: Seed.

Herbal Uses: The powdered seeds are taken in doses of one-fourth to one teaspoon to promote digestion and relieve gas. Caraway tea also relieves menstrual cramps, as it helps bring on the menstruation. Caraway increases breast milk. To make the tea, steep three teaspoons of the ground seeds in one-half cup of water for twenty minutes (use a kitchen blender to lightly crush the seed). Take up to one and a half cups a day in one-fourth cup doses, or simply chew the seeds. One to four drops of the essential oil may be taken as a digestive aid. For colicky babies, soak one ounce of the ground seed in a pint of cold water for about six hours. The dose is from one to three teaspoons of the infusion, or boil three teaspoons of seed in one-half cup of milk for a few minutes, then steep for ten minutes. The powdered seeds are moistened to make a poultice for bruises and earaches. Follow the usual directions for a poultice given on page 15.

Magical Uses: Caraway is often added to love potions to keep lovers from being unfaithful. The seeds are placed in poppets and used in spells to find one's mate. They are said to inspire lust when baked into cakes or breads. Put some in your wedding cake, or use it instead of rice to throw at the bride and groom. Pigeons are very fond of it too!

CORIANDER, *CORIANDRUM SATIVUM*

Parts Used: Seed and leaf.

Herbal Uses: The seeds are strengthening to the urinary system. The leaf and seed are infused to treat bladder infections. The tea helps with stomach problems such as gas and indigestion. Steep two teaspoons of the dried seed per cup of boiled water for twenty minutes, and take up to one cup a day. The powdered seed and the oil are used to flavor other herbal preparations and to ease griping in laxative formulas. Use one-fourth to one-half teaspoon at a time. Coriander is a common ingredient of Indian curries.

Magical Uses: The powdered seed is added to warm wine as a lust potion. Put some in the chalice for the ritual.

DAMIANA, *TURNERA APHRODISIACA*

Part Used: Leaf.

Herbal Uses: A classic aphrodisiac, damiana works by sending blood to the genital area, which the user interprets as being "turned on." It must be used consistently for several weeks before an effect is noticed. The leaf is infused to treat sexual trauma, frigidity, and impotence. It also clears the kidneys, helps the digestion, relieves constipation, and benefits lung problems and coughs. Steep two teaspoons of leaf per cup of water for twenty minutes. Take one-fourth cup four times a day.

Homeopathic Uses: Homeopaths use *Turnera* for impotency, nervous prostration that leads to sexual debility, incontinence in the aged, prostatic discharge, and menstrual irregularity in the young.

Magical Uses: Damiana is worn, burned, drunk, and carried to promote lust. It is especially potent when placed in something red.

ELDERFLOWER, *SAMBUCUS NIGRA*

Parts Used and Herbal Uses: Please see page 69 in "The Herbs of Meán Samhraidh."

Magical Uses: Elder leaves, flowers, and berries are used in wish-fulfillment rituals and to bring blessings and luck to a handfasted pair.

GINGER, *ZINGIBER OFFICINALIS*

Part Used: Root.

Herbal Uses: The root is warming to the body, is slightly antiseptic, and promotes internal secretions. Chop about two inches of the fresh root, cover with one cup of water, and simmer for about twenty minutes, or one-half teaspoon of the powdered root can be simmered in one cup of water. Add lemon juice, honey, and a slight pinch of cayenne. A few teaspoons of brandy will make an even more effective remedy for colds. This preparation treats fevers, chest colds, and flu. A bath or a foot-soak in hot ginger tea is also beneficial. The tea without additives helps indigestion, colic, diarrhea, and alcoholic gastritis. Dried ginger in capsules or in juice is taken to avoid carsickness and seasickness. Use about one-half teaspoon of the powder. It works well for dogs and children!

Homeopathic Uses: Homeopaths use *Zingiber* for weakness in the intestinal tract and in the reproductive system, kidneys, and lungs. It treats dry coughs and asthma that is worse in the morning and without anxiety. A peculiar symptom calling for the remedy is that the patient is worse when eating melons.

Magical Uses: Ginger enhances all spells, especially love spells, being a spicy and "hot" herb.

HOLLY, *ILEX AQUIFOLIUM*

Parts Used and Herbal Uses: Please see page 35 in"The Herbs of Meán Geimhridh."

Magical Uses: Traditional crowns for the bride and groom are made of holly (a male plant) and ivy (a female plant). Wreaths and altar decorations are made from these herbs as well.

IVY, *HEDERA* SPP.

Parts Used and Herbal Uses: Please see page 60 in "The Herbs of Beltaine."

Magical Uses: Ivy was once used to crown poets and, in ancient wedding rites, to crown the bride and groom (see "Holly," above). An early Christian church council attempted to ban the use of ivy in decorations because of its Pagan associations.

JASMINE, *JASMINUM OFFICINALE*

Parts Used and Herbal Uses: Please see page 51 in "The Herbs of Meán Earraigh."

Magical Uses: Jasmine flowers are added to the ritual cup to promote spiritual love and to draw wealth.

LAVENDER, *LAVANDULA VERA = L. OFFICINALIS*

Parts Used and Herbal Uses: Please see page 71 in "The Herbs of Meán Samhraidh."

Magical Uses: Lavender is worn, carried, and placed in the ritual cup. It is a classic ingredient of love spells, being especially attractive to men. Lavender, if worn, protects against abuse from a spouse.

LEMON VERBENA, *LIPPIA CITRIODORA = ALOYSIA CITRIODORA = VERBENA TRIPHYLLA*

Parts Used: Leaf and flowering top.

Herbal Uses: The leaves and flowering tops are used to lower fevers and to relieve gas and indigestion. Lemon verbena is calming, a sedative for the nerves. Steep two teaspoons per cup of water for twenty minutes and take one-fourth cup four times a day. Stimulating to the skin, lemon verbena makes a good facial scrub for pimples and blemishes. To make the scrub, grind the dry herb or use the powder and mix in a little natural clay and ground oatmeal.

Magical Uses: Lemon verbena in oil or incense is an herb of protection and purification. Worn on the person, it will make one attractive to the opposite sex. It is a common ingredient of love spells.

LICORICE, *GLYCYRRHIZA GLABRA*

Part Used: Root.

Herbal Uses: Licorice root has a special affinity for the lungs and the spleen. It is strengthening to the digestion and soothes duodenal ulcers. It is a good herb to improve energy. Coughs, colds, and asthma are soothed by it, as are sore throats and abdominal pains. As a plant, it seems to neutralize other plant poisons; hence, it is often added to formulas to arrest allergic reactions. Simmer one teaspoon of the root per cup of water for twenty minutes; take one-fourth cup four times a day. Licorice roots are chewed by those who are breaking the cigarette habit.

   CAUTION: *Persons with high blood pressure and edema should avoid it, as should women who experience a lot of water retention before the menses.*

Magical Uses: Licorice roots are chewed to increase sexual vitality. A magical herb suitable for making wands, it is frequently added to lust spells and love potions. Licorice brings fidelity and passion to a sexual union.

LOTUS, *NELUMBO NUCIFERA*

Parts Used and Herbal Uses: Please see page 154 in "Herbs for Funerals."

Magical Uses: Lotus antidotes love spells. As a general spiritual elixir, lotus is worn to bring the blessings of the gods.

MAPLE, *ACER* SPP.

Parts Used and Herbal Uses: Please see page 191 in "Baby Blessing Herbs."

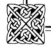

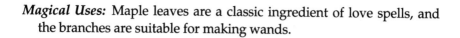

Magical Uses: Maple leaves are a classic ingredient of love spells, and the branches are suitable for making wands.

MARJORAM, *ORIGANUM MAJORANA*; WILD MARJORAM, *O. VULGARE*

Parts Used and Herbal Uses: Please see page 155 in "Herbs for Funerals."

Magical Uses: Marjoram is woven into the wedding wreath. It brings joy and is a common herb in love spells.

MEADOWSWEET, *SPIRAEA ULMARIA*

Parts Used and Herbal Uses: Please see page 98 in "Herbs of the Druids."

Magical Uses: Meadowsweet is an herb of happiness. An ingredient of love spells, its flowers are steeped in wine and herb beers. Place it in the bridal bouquet and in the chalice.

MISTLETOE, *VISCUM ALBUM*

Parts Used and Herbal Uses: Please see page 100 in "Herbs of the Druids."

Magical Uses: A few berries are placed in the chalice.

ORCHID ROOT (SATYRION ROOT), *ORCHIS* SPP.

Parts Used and Herbal Uses: Please see page 61 in "The Herbs of Beltaine."

Magical Uses: Orchid is a frequent ingredient in love spells and potions. Add the flowers to wreaths, crowns, and bouquets. Place some of the root in the chalice.

QUINCE, *CYDONIA VULGARIS = PYRUS CYDONIA*

Parts Used: Fruit and seed.

Herbal Uses: The sour fruit of the quince is high in vitamin C. It is simmered to make an antiinflammatory and pain-relieving tea for back pains, cramps, abdominal pains, spasms in the calves, ligament pains, and blood congestion. Use one or two fruits per cup of water; the dose is three to twelve grams (about 5 teaspoons). The fruit is high in tannic acid, and a syrup made from it will help with diarrhea. Follow the general directions for syrup on page 16. The seeds may be soaked in water until a mucilaginous mass appears. This can then be taken as a laxative or placed on the skin overnight to contract wrinkles.

Homeopathic Uses: Homeopaths use *Cydonia vulgaris* to strengthen the reproductive organs and the stomach.

Magical Uses: Quince is sacred to Venus/Aphrodite and, as an herb of love and happiness, is sent as a present to a bridal pair. Lovers may send gifts of quince to each other, and the fruit may be eaten by the bridal couple in the ceremony.

Quince is served to a "significant other" to ensure fidelity and to a pregnant woman to bring brilliance to her yet unborn child.

ROSE, *ROSA* SPP.

Parts Used and Herbal Uses: Please see page 51 in "The Herbs of Meán Earraigh."

Magical Uses: Red roses, symbols of passion, and pink roses, symbols of love, are used in all aspects of the ceremony. Strew them before the bridal pair, use them on the altar, wear them, and place them in the chalice and in the marriage bed.

ROSEMARY, *ROSEMARINUS OFFICINALIS*

Parts Used and Herbal Uses: Please see page 182 in "House Blessing Herbs."

Magical Uses: Rosemary is an herb of consecration and remembrance. It is added to incense, placed in the chalice, and distributed to guests.

SKULLCAP, *SCUTELLARIA GALERICULATA*, *S. LATERIFLORA*

Scutellaria galericulata is a European variety; *S. lateriflora* is the American species.

Parts Used: Whole herb.

Herbal Uses: Skullcap has a special affinity for the nervous system. Con-

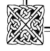

vulsions, hysteria, headache, and insomnia are treated with this plant. It is reputed to be a cure for rabies and has been used in epilepsy. Skullcap is a useful brain tonic, especially when combined with lady's slipper, valerian, and passion flower. It is used to help in alcohol and drug withdrawal and strengthens meditation.

Homeopathic Uses: Homeopaths use *Scutellaria lateriflora* for conditions of nervous fear, cardiac irritability, spasms, muscular twitching, and frontal headaches. Nightmares, migraine with aching eyeballs, nausea, colic, and diarrhea are within its sphere, as is impotency with a terror of never getting better.

Magical Uses: Skullcap is added to the chalice as a strengthener of vows. It is given to one's spouse to wear as protection from the charms of the opposite sex.

YARROW, *ACHILLEA MILLEFOLIUM*

Parts Used: Above-ground portions of the herb.

Herbal Uses: This is a classic herb for flu, especially the intestinal variety. Try a mixture of elderflower, peppermint, and yarrow to bring down a fever and induce perspiration. The tea benefits the kidneys. Yarrow is used in salves for hemorrhoids and in poultices to stop bleeding and help heal wounds. Cramps and rheumatism are treated with the tea, as are intestinal gas, diarrhea, anorexia, and hyperacidity.

Homeopathic Uses: Homeopaths use *Millefolium* for hemorrhages with bright red blood, hernia, bad effects from falls or overlifting, and continued high temperatures; it is a classic treatment for nosebleed, bloody urine, bleeding from the bowels, bloody coughs, and profuse menses with bright red blood.

Magical Uses: A common herb in love spells, yarrow is included in wedding decorations and hung over the bridal bed. Large patches of yarrow growing in a field indicate a very grounded energy spot. Sit there to center and relax.

CHAPTER 16

Ꮋome, a Ꮋaven of Peace and Prosperity

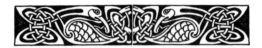

> And thou, Waybroad! [plantain]
> Mother of Worts
> Open from eastward
> Mighty within;
> Over thee carts creaked,
> Over thee queens rode,
> Over thee brides bridalled,
> Over thee bulls breathed.
> And these thou withstoodst
> Venom and all vile things
> And all loathely ones
> That through the land rove.
>
> *Aelfic (11th century)*

> O who can tell
> The hidden power of herbes and might of Magick spell?"
>
> *Edmund Spenser,* **The Faerie Queene**

The east is the direction to invoke for house blessings. Anyone who has traveled in Ireland* will appreciate the mystical association of the east

---

* Ireland is frequently alluded to because it is the most Celtic of countries. The ancient Romans never managed to get there, and its original culture remained intact for a longer period than other Celtic societies enjoyed.

with wealth, householding, beautiful clothes, abundance, and hospitality. The moist and verdant quality of eastern hills and valleys is the perfect inspiration for prosperity rituals.

The west is associated with teaching, history-keeping, eloquence, and judgements; the north with battles, pride, the Gods, and the fires of conflict and of the spirit. The south is the home of music, subtle arts, poetry, and waterfalls—a Goddess direction. The center holds the qualities of leadership, fame, dignity and stability.*

Inhospitality is one of the gravest reproaches to be held against a Druid or a Celt. The visiting stranger is felt to be almost sacred—who can say whether the stranger is a God or Goddess in disguise?

Hospitality extends to the fairy realm as well. After a ritual, a gift of spirits, a plate of food, or a bowl of milk is left at the western side of the house for the fairies' pleasure. And one should never make an addition to the western side of the home without first consulting the fairies. To do this, one must cut a piece of turf and leave it upside down overnight. If by the next morning the sod has not been turned back, one has their tacit approval for the addition.

House Blessing Herbs

Basil, Bay Laurel, Camphor, Cinquefoil, Cowslip, Elderflower, Figwort, Garlic, Juniper, Mandrake, Melilot, Pine, Plantain, Rosemary, Rowan, Rue

Please refer to chapter 2, "Herbal Basics," for methods of preparation.

Basil, Ocimum basilicum

Parts Used and Herbal Uses: Please see page 41 in "The Herbs of Imbolc/Oimealg."

Magical Uses: Basil is used in rites of exorcism and to bring happiness to the home. Burn it as incense, sew it into sachets, weave it into wreaths, or sprinkle the powder in the corners of rooms.

---

*Please see "Sacred Groves and Circles" for a fuller evocation of the directional correspondences.

BAY LAUREL, *LAURUS NOBILIS*

Parts Used and Herbal Uses: Please see page 33 in "The Herbs of Meán Geimhridh."

Magical Uses: Bay leaves are carried or placed around the home to ward off illness and hexes.

CAMPHOR, *CINNAMOMUM CAMPHORA*

Parts Used: Crystallized extract and leaf.

Herbal Uses: Both the leaf and the crystallized extract are used for wet lung conditions such as asthma and bronchitis. Camphor is useful in depression, exhaustion, and stomach cramps, and to improve circulation. Use about two teaspoons of leaf per cup of water and steep for twenty minutes. Take one-fourth cup four times a day. Alternatively, use one teaspoon of the crystallized extract per two cups of water. Take it in one-teaspoon doses four times a day. The tincture is also available and is used in doses of five to ten drops four times a day. Camphor is incorporated into salves for external use to kill parasites and treat ringworm, scabies, and itch. See the instructions for salves given on page 14. The oil opens the lungs, making breathing easier, and helps with muscular and joint pain, arthritis, and bruises (*not* for open wounds). The salve functions as a "smelling salt," and the herb has been used internally to revive those in coma or delirium. Camphor can be burned to purify the air or inhaled to open lung passages.

    CAUTION: *Do not use this herb if you are pregnant or if you are very weak and debilitated. Only natural plant extracts should be used, as chemical camphor is contaminated with industrial poisons.*

Homeopathic Uses: Homeopaths use *Camphora* for states of collapse in which the body is icy cold. It is a classic remedy for cholera and for the first stages of a cold, violent convulsions, and insomnia. Herbal camphor antidotes homeopathic remedies, and this should be remembered if you are attempting to combine it with anything else!

Magical Uses: Burn camphor in the home to purify the air and to dispel disease.

CINQUEFOIL, *POTENTILLA REPTANS*, *POTENTILLA CANADENSIS*

Parts Used and Herbal Uses: Please see page 48 in "The Herbs of Meán Earraigh."

Magical Uses: Drain an egg by pricking a hole in both ends of the egg and blowing out the yolk. Fill the eggshell with cinquefoil, tape it shut, and hide it somewhere in the home as an herb of protection.

COWSLIP (PRIMROSE), *PRIMULA VERIS*, *P. OFFICINALIS*

Parts Used: Leaves, flowers, and root.

Herbal Uses: The flowers are used in salves for sunburn and dry skin. The leaves are used in wound poultices. Follow the guidelines for salves and poultices given on pages 14 and 15. Two teaspoons of the dried flowers taken as tea prevent migraine, insomnia, and night-mares. Steep two teaspoons of the flowers in one cup of water for twenty minutes. Take one-fourth cup four times a day. Make a fresh batch every day. The dried root is simmered for its expectorant prop-erties. Simmer two teaspoons of root in one cup of water for twenty minutes. Take one-fourth cup four times a day. Primrose benefits bronchitis and whooping cough. It is a "blood cleanser" and useful for gouty or rheumatic conditions. The herb or root can be tinctured following the guidelines on page 15. The dose is five to twenty drops four times a day.

> CAUTION: *Some people are allergic to primroses.*

Homeopathic Uses: Homeopaths use *Primula veris* for neuralgia, mi-graine, vertigo, rheumatic pain, and gout. A strange "leading" symp-tom is that the urine smells of violets.

Magical Uses: Cowslip is hidden in the front of the house to discourage unwanted visitors.

ELDERFLOWER, *SAMBUCUS NIGRA*

Parts Used and Herbal Uses: Please see page 69 in "The Herbs of Meán Samhraidh."

Magical Uses: Elder is an herb of blessing, consecration, and wish ful-fillment. The flowers, leaves, or berries can be strewn on a person, place, or thing.

FIGWORT, *SCROPHULARIA NODOSA*

Parts Used and Herbal Uses: Please see page 92 in "Herbs of the Druids."

Magical Uses: Figwort is smoked over the Midsummer fire and hung in the home or worn as an amulet of protection.

GARLIC, *ALLIUM SATIVA*

Part Used: Bulb.

Herbal Uses: The garlic bulb is one of the great herbal "polycrests"— herbs of many uses. Fresh garlic is a preventative and a cure for intestinal worms. It is generally taken in one-teaspoon doses, three to six times a day, with some grated fresh ginger root. Garlic is a natural antibiotic for internal and external use. Mash it and use it as a wound dressing. Internally, it kills staphylococcus, streptococcus, salmonella, and *Candida albicans*. For a sore throat, lightly roast unpeeled cloves in a dry frying pan, peel them when they grow soft, and eat them. For pinworms, a slightly smashed fresh clove can be inserted into the rectum with olive oil. For vaginal infections, smash a few cloves and wrap them in cheese cloth. Insert directly into the vagina. Fresh raw garlic is more effective than the powdered and extracted forms available for sale. Garlic has been shown to be more effective than tetracycline as an antibiotic.

    CAUTION: *Pregnant women and persons with "hot and fiery" temperaments should avoid overuse of garlic.*

Homeopathic Uses: Homeopaths use *Allium sativum* for colitis, tuberculosis, painful constipation, bronchitis, painful breasts, and skin eruptions during the menses. The remedy is more effective for meat eaters than for exclusive vegetarians.

Magical Uses: In the home, braids of garlic guard against evil, repel thieves, and turn away the envious. And of course, garlic protects against vampires. It is a very effective blessing for new homes.

JUNIPER, *JUNIPERUS COMMUNIS*

Parts Used and Herbal Uses: Please see page 36 in "The Herbs of Meán Geimhridh."

Magical Uses: Juniper is used to ritually sweep out the rooms of a new home or when purification is desired.

MANDRAKE, *MANDRAGORA OFFICINALIS*

Parts Used and Herbal Uses: Please see page 95 in "Herbs of the Druids."

Magical Uses: Mandrake is placed on the mantle. It is soaked in water, which is then sprinkled around the home to bring joy and prosperity.

MELILOT, *MELILOTUS OFFICINALIS, MELILOTUS ALBA*

Part Used: Flowering herb.

Herbal Uses: Yellow melilot is used in poultices and salves for boils, swellings, arthritis, rheumatism, and headaches. To make a poultice put one-half ounce of the dried plant in a cloth bag, boil for one minute in water, steep for three minutes, and apply as hot as can be borne. To make the salve, follow the general instructions given on page 14. The tea is used to wash sores and wounds and as an antiin-flammatory eye wash. Internally, it helps bronchitis, insomnia, neural-gia, stomach upset, and colic. Steep one teaspoon of herb per cup of water for twenty minutes. Take up to one and a half cups a day. For headaches and joint pains, try making melilot into an herb pillow. White melilot (M. alba) is used in the same way.

 CAUTION: *This plant contains coumarin and is an anticoagulant. It should be avoided by those who bleed easily and by anyone about to undergo surgery. Large doses can produce vomiting.*

Homeopathic Uses: Homeopaths use *Melilotus* (yellow melilot or sweet clover) for hemorrhages, headaches, infantile spasms, epilepsy from a blow to the head, and joint pain. All symptoms are worse during rainy weather or approaching storms and at 4:00 P.M.

Magical Uses: Melilot is an herb of protection when hung in the house, car, or barn.

PINE, *PINUS* SPP.

Parts Used and Herbal Uses: Please see page 37 in "The Herbs of Meán Geimhridh."

Magical Uses: Pine is hung in the home to bring joy, and burned to bring peace and purification.

PLANTAIN, *PLANTAGO LANCEOLATA, P. MAJOR, P. MEDIA*

Part Used: Leaf.

Herbal Uses: Ribwort, or the lance-leaf plantain (*P. lanceolata*), is especially suitable for lung and throat problems, especially when there is mucous congestion. A tea of the dried leaf helps coagulate blood. Steep two teaspoons of herb per cup of water for twenty minutes and take up to one and a half cups a day in one-fourth cup doses, unsweetened. The juice of the fresh plant helps with gastrointestinal problems: one tablespoon of the fresh juice is taken in water or milk three times a day. The fresh leaves are used in poultices for insect bites, wounds, and hemorrhoids. Follow the directions for poultices given on page 15. Plantago major, the broad-leaved plantain, is used in the same way, and its juice also relieves bladder problems and stomach ulcers. The tea of the leaf is used in douches. Plantain poultices are very effective for wound healing; adding a pinch of cayenne pepper will encourage embedded material such as glass and splinters to emerge. Plantago media, the woolly plantain, is used the same way as the others.

Homeopathic Uses: Homeopaths use *Plantago major* for earache, toothache, and eye pain due to tooth decay or ear infection. Pyorrhea, depression, and insomnia are treated by it. It causes an aversion to tobacco—smoke addicts take note! The tincture is applied locally to toothache, otorrhea, pruritus, incised wounds, and poison-oak.

Magical Uses: Plantain is hung in the home and the car as an herb of protection.

ROSEMARY, *ROSEMARINUS OFFICINALIS*

Parts Used: Leaf and flower.

Herbal Uses: The leaf and flowers are stimulating to the liver and the digestion. For this reason, rosemary is a classic herb for migraine headache when associated with liver or stomach torpidity. Rosemary increases the circulation and slightly raises blood pressure. To make the tea, steep two teaspoons of the dried flowering tops in one cup of water for twenty minutes. Take one-fourth cup four times a day. Use rosemary in salves for eczema, wounds, and sores. Follow the general directions given for salves on page 14. The tea makes a mouthwash for bad breath. The oil benefits stomach and nerves. Steep the herb in white wine for a week and strain. Rub the rosemary wine into gouty or paralyzed limbs. Taken internally, the wine quiets the heart and stimulates the kidneys, brain, and nervous system. Rosemary tea relieves depression. Rosemary and coltsfoot are smoked as herbal tobacco to relieve asthma and lung conditions.

CAUTION: *When rosemary is used as a tea, the dose should not exceed one cup per day. Overdose can cause fatal poisoning.*

Homeopathic Uses: Homeopaths use *Rosemarinus* for conditions of premature menstruation, violent pains followed by uterine hemorrhage, a feeling of heaviness and drowsiness in the head, chills, icy coldness in the lower extremities, and thirstlessness followed by heat.

Magical Uses: As an herb of purification, rosemary can be a substitute for frankincense. "Any home where rosemary thrives is a home where the mistress rules." Rosemary or rosemary with juniper berries is burned as a protection from disease. Place it in books and drawers to repel moths.

ROWAN, *SORBUS AUCUPARIA*

Parts Used and Herbal Uses: Please see page 62 in "The Herbs of Beltaine."

Magical Uses: Rowan is an herb of protection in the home. Make small, equal-armed crosses with its wood, sew it into sachets, or weave wreaths of it as house decorations.

RUE, *RUTA GRAVEOLENS*

Parts Used and Herbal Uses: Please see page 160 in "Herbs for Funerals."

Magical Uses: Rue is burned, strewn into corners, and used to asperge the house as an herb of purification and to cancel negativity.

CHAPTER 17

From Childbirth to Puberty and Initiation

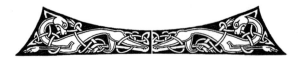

Every night and every morn
Some to misery are born.
Every morn and every night
Some are born to sweet delight.
Some are born to sweet delight,
Some are born to endless night.

We are led to believe a lie
When we see *with*, not *through*, the eye,
Which was born in a night, to perish in a night,
When the soul slept in beams of light.

William Blake, "Auguries of Innocence"

I have no name;
I am but two days old.
What shall I call thee?
I happy am,
Joy is my name.
Sweet joy befall thee!

William Blake, "Infant Joy"

Childhood is a special time marked by the ritual phases of naming, puberty, and initiation. But before the cycle of life can begin, the fertility of the mother must be assured. Several ancient rituals still survive that can be used to alter infertility. If we contemplate the powerful effects of self-hypnosis, guided imagery, and mental attitude on diseases such as cancer, we can begin to appreciate the worth of the following practices.

An old Scottish rite involves placing a quartz pebble shaped like an egg into water taken from a running stream. A woman desiring children washes her feet in the water. In County Mayo, Ireland, barren women walk seven times around a "bed"—a depression in the Earth at a location used by women for countless generations. They then enter the "bed" and turn around seven times. Upon leaving, they pick up some small pebbles to take home. Some women choose to sleep in the bed for a night. Sitting on a magic stone is said to bring fertility to a barren woman. A woman may spend the night in the cleft of a rock to help ensure pregnancy. Drinking the dew that collects in a stone is said to do the same.

Forked carrots are potent fertility symbols, and gifts of bunches of carrots may be presented to women and men who wish to conceive. Nuts, especially acorns, are helpful in enhancing fertility as well. A bride may gather wheat straws for the boys she wishes to conceive and oat straws for the girls she hopes to bear and weave them into a garter. (Apparently, this charm is only effective for virgins, and the garter must stay in place from Friday until Monday without breaking.)

Wells are known as secret entrances to the Otherworld and the Earth Mother. In one traditional fertility ritual, women join hands and dance in a circle. The eldest woman sits in the center, dipping water from the well and sprinkling it on the others.

The Earth Mother is also seen as a help to the woman in labor, should she lie directly on the ground to draw the Earth's strength in her time of travail. (Pregnant women can pull bits of clothing through a hole in a stone to ensure a speedy labor.) Herbs which have grown rooted in the Earth ease the stages of labor, stimulate the wearied muscles and will, and guard mother and child against blood loss and infection.

Once the child is born, the umbilical cord is hung in a sacred tree, usually a hawthorn. (Animal placentas are hung there, also, when the domestic beasts give birth.)

The first important ritual in a child's life is the naming ceremony. This rite celebrates the child's death to the spirit world and rebirth into the world of mortals. After this ritual, the child is officially "present" on the Earth, since before the ritual it was still partly in the Otherworld. The sacred element of water is used to symbolize a ceremonial birth that introduces the child to the ritual cycles of the sacred Earth year. The ritual is significant for the parents as well, because it is here that they are initiated into the spiritual and mundane responsibilities of parenthood. A tree is often planted to mark the occasion.

The next important childhood rite is the puberty ceremony. This ritual marks the official beginning of separation from parents and the first phase of independent adult life. A new name, the acquisition of arms, victory over a symbolic or animal opponent, endurance tests, athletic contests, and music and poetry competitions typically mark the event.

A common theme is the entry into the land of shadow, where secret instructions are given and ordeals are assigned. The candidate may be instructed to spend time among graves, caves, or burial chambers and to return "reborn" to the sun's light. Hair-cutting is a traditional mark of initiation, as is the appearance of a mysterious male or female with whom sexual union is undertaken.

Later initiations involve "marrying" one's craft and symbolic union with the land, with the elements (earth, air, fire, and water), or with one's spiritual group. Surprise, confusion, and eventual triumph are the hallmarks of these rites. By far the greatest emphasis is on the liberation of the initiate through victory over fear and a widening of the boundaries of spirit.

Baby Blessing Herbs

Arborvitae (Yellow Cedar), Ash, Birch, Daisy, Elderflower, Elecampane, Elm, Flax, Hawthorn, Holly, Iris, Maple, Milkweed, Mulberry, Lavender, Parsley, Rosemary, Unicorn Root

Please refer to chapter 2, "Herbal Basics," for methods of preparation.

Arborvitae (Yellow Cedar), *Thuja occidentalis*

Parts Used and Herbal Uses: Please see page 25 in "The Herbs of Samhain."

Magical Uses: Arborvitae, the "Tree of Life," is burned in baby blessing rituals and is used as a decoration to bring long life and even immortality to the child.

ASH, *FRAXINUS EXCELSIOR, F. AMERICANA*

Parts Used and Herbal Uses: Please see page 33 in "The Herbs of Meán Geimhridh."

Magical Uses: Burying a newborn's first nail trimmings under an ash ensures the child will grow up a good singer. Sick children are passed through a cleft in an ash sapling to effect a cure.

BIRCH, *BETULA ALBA, B. LUTEA, B. LENTA*

Parts Used: Leaf, bark, and twig.

Herbal Uses: The white birch makes a leaf tea that dissolves kidney stones if taken over a long time. Steep two teaspoons of leaf per cup of water for twenty minutes. The dose is one to one and a half cups over a day. Birch twigs and leaves are simmered and added to bath water for itchy skin conditions and falling hair. Taken before bed, the tea is sedative. The young shoots and leaves make a tonic laxative. The inner bark is simmered and used in fevers. Twigs and bark are simmered using two teaspoons of plant per cup of water for twenty minutes. The dose is one-fourth cup taken four times a day. The twigs of *B. lutea* (yellow birch) and *B. lenta* (black birch) are gathered in spring and simmered gently for twenty minutes to make a delicious beverage. Please note: the leaves must be used fresh, and not after Midsummer, as they will then contain natural insecticides. The white birch has no real flavor and does not make a good beverage tea.

Magical Uses: Birch is a feminine tree and an embodiment of the Great Mother. Cradles are often made of her wood as a protection for the child.

DAISY, *BELLIS PERENNIS*

Part Used: Above-ground portions of the herb.
This is not to be confused with the common American oxeye daisy, *Chrysanthemum leucanthemum.*

Herbal Uses: The English daisy as an herb is a gentle laxative. To make a tea, steep one tablespoon of the herb per cup of water for twenty minutes. Take up to one cup a day in one-fourth cup doses. The fresh flowers are used in poultices for burns, injuries, and inflammations.

Follow the standard directions for poultices and salves given on pages 14 and 15. Lung conditions, colds, sluggish digestion, gas, colic, and liver, kidney, and bladder problems benefit from it. The wild English daisy can be used internally and externally at the same time for maximum relief.

Homeopathic Uses: Homeopaths use *Bellis perennis* after surgery and for muscular soreness, lameness, mechanical injuries, sprains and bruises, trauma to the pelvic region, inability to walk during pregnancy, and boils.

Magical Uses: Known as "bairnwort" in Scotland because children use it to make daisy chains; daisy is an appropriate herb to decorate the cradle and the altar.

ELDERFLOWER, *SAMBUCUS NIGRA*

Parts Used and Herbal Uses: Please see page 69 in "The Herbs of Meán Samhraidh."

Magical Uses: To bring the blessings of the Eldermother, a bath for the rite is prepared of elderflower water. Elder is burned in her honor as incense.

ELECAMPANE (ELFWORT, SCABWORT), *INULA HELENIUM*

Part Used: Root.

Herbal Uses: The autumn-dug root is excellent for coughs and has been used by Native American healers to cure tuberculosis. All chronic lung conditions such as bronchitis and asthma are helped by it. It is generally mixed with other lung herbs. Elecampane produces an active principle called helenin, which is antiseptic and antibacterial, making the root useful in salves and surgical dressings.

Homeopathic Uses: Homeopaths use *Inula* for diabetes, bronchial infections, and "bearing down" sensations in the pelvic region with labor-like pains.

Magical Uses: Elecampane is burned as incense to bring joy and is worn to attract love.

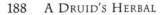

ELM, *ULMUS CAMPESTRIS, U. FULVA*

Parts Used: Bark and leaf.

Herbal Uses: The dried inner bark of *Ulmus campestris* (common elm) has been used both internally and externally for ringworm. The bark of young branches is made into a tea for herpes, itch, scurf, and other skin ailments. To make the tea, simmer two teaspoons of bark or twigs per cup of water for twenty minutes. Take one-fourth cup four times a day. The bark and leaf are tinctured in vinegar to make a skin wash. Follow the general directions for tinctures given on page 15. *U. fulva*, the slippery elm, has a soothing, mucilaginous inner bark that is used externally in poultices for wounds and inflammations (simply add water to the dried and powdered bark until it has a pie-dough consistency, and apply). As a tea, it is used for sore throats, bronchitis, diarrhea, urinary problems, and dysentery. It is incorporated into suppositories, enemas, and douches because of its soothing nature. Experience has taught me that only *very small* amounts of the powdered bark can be added to a douche or a tea. It gels quickly into a mass, so be watchful and put in only a teaspoon at a time.

    CAUTION: *Elm trees have been much depleted by Dutch elm disease. Use only the bark of outer twigs to avoid harming the tree.*

Magical Uses: Slippery elm is hung around a child's neck to ensure speaking skills in later life.

FLAX (LINSEED), *LINUM USITATISSIMUM*

Part Used: Seed.

Herbal Uses: A teaspoon of the seed is placed in a quart of water and gently simmered down to one-half quart. The resulting liquid is given for constipation, for ulcerated sore throat, and as an expectorant for bronchitis in one-fourth cup doses throughout the day. To pass a gallstone, take one and a half to two tablespoons of linseed oil and lie on your left side for a half hour. The whole seeds (about two tablespoons) can be taken with plenty of water to relieve constipation. Follow with stewed prunes or prune juice. The cooked seeds are added to fresh grated carrots, and the mix is warmed to make a poultice for rheumatism and swellings.

Homeopathic Uses: Homeopaths use *Linum usitatissimum* as a poultice for asthma and hives. As a decoction it treats cystitis, asthma, hay fever, nettle rash, and paralysis of the tongue.

Magical Uses: The child who runs or dances in a flax field at the age of seven is assured of growing up to be attractive. Newborn babies are placed in a flax field to sleep for similar reasons.

HAWTHORN, *CRATEGUS* SPP.

Parts Used and Herbal Uses: Please see page 59 in "The Herbs of Beltaine."

Magical Uses: Hawthorn is placed in a child's cradle to shield it from evil spells.

HOLLY, *ILEX AQUIFOLIUM*

Parts Used and Herbal Uses: Please see page 35 in "The Herbs of Meán Geimhridh."

Magical Uses: An infusion of holly is sprinkled on the newborn child as an herb of protection.

IRIS, *IRIS VERSICOLOR*

Parts Used and Herbal Uses: Please see page 43 in "The Herbs of Imbolc/Oimealg."

Magical Uses: Iris brings wisdom, faith, courage, and joy. Plant some on the day of the baby blessing as a gift for the newborn as she or he grows.

LAVENDER, *LAVANDULA VERA = L. OFFICINALIS*

Parts Used and Herbal Uses: Please see page 71 in "The Herbs of Meán Samhraidh."

Magical Uses: Lavender is burned during childbirth and labor as an herb of peace and tranquility. The joyful scent of lavender is welcome at baby blessing rituals.

Maple, *Acer* spp.

Parts Used: Bark, sap, and leaves.

Herbal Uses: Calcium, necessary for bones, teeth, blood-clotting, healthy muscles and nerves, enzymatic processes, and fluid secretions, is found in abundance in maple syrup. Iron to build red blood cells is found in smaller but significant amounts. Maple syrup is a good sugar substitute, being less sweet and having more yang qualities. The bark of *Acer rubrum*, the red maple, is simmered to make an eyewash. To make the tea, simmer two teaspoons of bark per cup of water and strain carefully through a cheesecloth or coffee filter to protect the eyes. The immature leaves of maple are edible in the early spring. Two tablespoons of maple syrup, the juice of a half lemon, and a pinch of cayenne pepper, taken with eight ounces of water several times a day, makes a good fasting beverage to clear the body of toxins.

Magical Uses: To help a child achieve a long life, pass it ritually through the branches of a maple tree.

Milkweed, *Asclepias syriaca*

Parts Used and Herbal Uses: Please see page 86 in "The Herbs of Meán Fómhair."

Magical Uses: The juice of milkweed bestows health, long life, and immortality. Use a few drops to anoint a new baby.
  CAUTION: *The juice is not to be taken internally!*

Mulberry, *Morus rubra*, M. *alba*, M. *nigra*

Parts Used: Root, twig, leaf, and berry.

Herbal Uses: Morus rubra, the red mulberry, is an American tree. The bark of the root is a remedy for tapeworms and a gentle laxative. Half a teaspoon of the powdered root can be taken with water for laxative effects, or two teaspoons of the bark can be simmered in one cup of water for twenty minutes and taken in quarter-cup doses as needed, up to one cup a day. The juice of the leaf was used by Native Americans to treat ringworm on the scalp. *M. nigra*, the black mulberry, a European tree, is used similarly. The bark of the root of *M. nigra* is used for tapeworm. Mulberries are made into drinks or fed whole to persons with fever. *M. alba* is a Chinese variety grown as an ornamental in the United States. The small branches of this tree are made into a decoction for rheumatic and arthritic pains. Simmer two teaspoons of the twigs per cup of water for twenty minutes and take quarter-cup doses, up to one cup a day. The fruit of *M. alba* is a blood tonic for anemia, debilitating diseases, vertigo, premature graying of the hair, and sleeplessness. It helps with constipation in the aged. The leaf of *M. alba* treats colds, fevers, and influenza when taken as tea. Steep two teaspoons of leaf in one cup of water and take one-fourth cup four times a day. The bark of the root is antiinflammatory to the lungs in cases of asthma, bronchitis, and wheezing and is especially useful when there is fever, thirst, and swelling of the extremities. Simmer two teaspoons of root bark in one cup of water for twenty minutes and take one-fourth cup four times a day.

CAUTION: *Avoid this plant if diarrhea or digestive weakness is present.*

Magical Uses: Mulberry is a magical tree of protection. Place the wood or a leaf somewhere near baby's cradle.

PARSLEY, *CARUM PETROSELINUM, PETROSELINUM SATIVUM*

Parts Used and Herbal Uses: Please see page 156 in "Herbs for Funerals." Expectant mothers should eat parsley and watercress during the pregnancy to keep the liver and kidneys strong. A bath in parsley tea is recommended before labor (and before rituals in general).

Magical Uses: Parsley is used in decorations for baby blessing rites.

ROSEMARY, *ROSEMARINUS OFFICINALIS*

Parts Used and Herbal Uses: Please see page 182 in "House Blessing Herbs."

Magical Uses: As an herb of consecration and of purification from disease, rosemary is a good choice for incense at a baby blessing.

Unicorn Root, *Chamaelirium luteum, Helonias diocia, Aletris farinosa*

Part Used: Root.

Herbal Uses: *Chamaelirium luteum*, the "false unicorn root," is used to enhance fertility. Many female problems are addressed by it, especially when there is a sensation of dragging in the abdomen, irregular menstruation, miscarriage, and morning sickness. It is tonic to the liver, kidney, and genitourinary tract. Digestive problems, back pains, and impotence are helped by it. Simmer two teaspoons of root in one cup of water for twenty minutes and take one-fourth cup four times a day. The tincture can be made according to the directions found on page 15 and taken in doses of five to fifteen drops with water, four times a day. Taken internally or applied externally in salves, false unicorn root removes worms and parasites. See page 14 for directions on how to make salves. *Aletris farinosa*, the "true unicorn root," is dried to make a stomach tonic for gas, colic, and indigestion and also a general tonic for the female reproductive tract. It also prevents miscarriage. Simmer two teaspoons of root per cup of water for twenty minutes and take one-fourth cup four times a day.

Homeopathic Uses: Homeopaths use *Aletris farinosa* (stargrass, true unicorn root) for anemia, exhaustion, premature and painful menstruation, prolapse of the uterus, and morning sickness. *Helonias-Chamaelirium* (unicorn root) is used for pelvic weakness with a dragging sensation and exhaustion, for "melancholy," lower back pain with kidney involvement, and suppressed menstruation. All symptoms are better when mental diversion is offered.

Magical Uses: Unicorn root is an herb of protection for baby and mother. It is worn as an amulet or carried in power bundles for this purpose.

APPENDIX A

Pronunciation Guide

Gaelic word	Pronounced as
Aillill	AL-ill
Agni	AHG-nee
Aengus Óg	ENG-us OAG
Argatlam	AHR-gat-lahv
Badbh	Boyv
Bean-drui	BEN-druee
Beltaine	BYAL-te-nye
Bíle	BEE-Lah
Boand	BOH-ahn
Brideóga	BREE-joag-a
Brighid	Breej
Bruig na Boinne	Brew na BO-IN-yeh
Caer Arianrhod	Kweer Ah-reean-ROAD
Caer Ibormeith	Kweer EE-vor-meh
Cailleach	KYE-lyakh
Celtic	KEL-tick
Cill Dara	Kill-DAHra
Cúchulainn	Coo-KHULL-in

Dagda	DOG-da
Danu	DAH-nuh
Deosil	JESH-eil
Diancecht	Jee-an KYEKHT
Duir	Dur
Éire	AIR-uh
Eochaid Ollathair	O-khi d OL-ather
Fionn	Finn *or* Fyoon
Glasen	GLOSS-un
Gorsedd	GORE-sedh
Gwydion	GWID-eon
Imbolc	Ih-mulk
Iníonacha an Daghdha	Een-eeohn-Ah ahn DOG-da
In Ruad Ró-fhessa	In ROO-ahd roo-AHssa
La Tene	Lah-TEN
Lleu	Lhoy
Loch	Lokh
Lubgort	LUV-ghort
Lugh	Loo
Lugnasad	LOO-nass-ah
Lugh Samildinach	Loo Sahv-il-DAWN-akh
Lungait	LUN-getch
Mabinogion	Mah-bin-OHG-yon
Maeldúin	Mweel-DOON
Manannán Mac Lir	MON-an-awn mock-lirr
Meán Earraigh	Myawn AR-ee
Meán Fómhair	Myawn FOE-wir
Meán Geimhridh	Myawn GEV-ree
Meán Samhraidh	Myawn SOUR-ee
Nemain	NYA-win
Nuada Argatlam	NOOa-dha AHR-gat-lahv

Oengus (Aengus)	ENG-us
Ogham	OH-ahm
Oimealg	OEE-MEHLG
Ollam	OL-lav
Roid	Royd
Samhain	SOW-in
Segais	SHAY-gesh
Sídhe	Shee
Sraif	Shrav
Táiltean	TAWL-chun
Táiltiu	TAWL-chuh
Táin Bó Cualinge	TAW-in bo COO-ill-na
Taranis	Tah-RAHnis
Tír na nOg	CHEER nah NOHG
Tír Tairngire	Cheer-TAR-gear-ah
Tuatha Dé Danann	Too-ha deh DON-awn
Uisneach	ISH-nyakh
Yggdrasil	IGG-dra-sill

APPENDIX B

Resources

For information on the Druid path—lessons by correspondence, quarterly journal, and initiations—write to Keltria, P.O. Box 48369 Minneapolis, MN 55448

HOMEOPATHY

For a directory of practitioners, study groups, and courses:

Boericke and Tafel
1011 Arch Street
Philadelphia, PA 19107
1-800-272-2820

The National Center for Homeopathy
801 North Fairfax Street, Suite 306
Alexandria, VA 22314
(703) 548-7790
FAX (703) 548-7792
E-mail nch (HomeoNet),
nch@igc.apc.org

Homeopathy Overnight Inc.
Order remedies seven days a week
(B&T, Dolisos, or Standard, all
common potencies)
1-800-Arnica30
FAX 1-800-456-1223

Standard Homeopathic Co.
210 W. 131st Street
Box 61067
Los Angeles, CA 90061

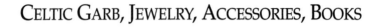

CELTIC GARB, JEWELRY, ACCESSORIES, BOOKS

Celtic Folkworks
R.D. 4 Box 210
Willow Grove Road
Newfield, NJ 08344
(609) 691-5968

David Morgan
(Welsh Clothing, Books, and
Accessories)
11812 North Creek Parkway N.
Suite 103
Bothell, WA 98011
1-800-324-4934

MAGICAL SUPPLIES

Abramelin Ritual Artisans
(Rare books, custom jewelry, and
magical tools)
124 Baptist Hill Road
Palmer, MA 01069
(413) 283-6502

Abyss
R.R. 1 Box 213
Chester, MA 01011
(413) 623-2155
FAX (413) 623-2156

Magus Books and Supplies
18305 20th Avenue North
Plymouth, MN 55447
(612) 379-7669

White Light Pentacles
P.O. Box 8163
Salem, MA 01971-8163
(Wholesale only)
1-800-MASTERY

HERBS

The American Herbalists Guild
P.O. Box 1683
Soquel, CA 95073
(408) 464-2441

Northeast Herb Association
(Catalog of practitioners, educators,
and growers)
P.O. Box 146
Marshfield, VT 05658-0146

Seeds of Change
(Rare and endangered vegetable and
medicinal plant seeds)
P.O. Box 15700
Santa Fe, NM 87506-5700

SUPPLIES

Herbalist and Alchemist Inc.
(Western and Chinese Herbs)
P.O. Box 553
Broadway, NJ 08808
(908) 689-9020

Mountain Rose Herbs
P.O. Box 2000
Redway, CA 95560
(800) 879-3337

Penn Herb Co. Ltd.
603 North Second Street
Philadelphia, PA 19123-3098

St. Johns Herb Garden, Inc.
7711 Hillmeade Rd.
Bowie, MD 20720
(301) 262-5302
FAX (301) 262-2489

BiBLioGRaphy

HISTORY AND LITERATURE

Bord, Janet, and Colin Bord. *Earth Rites*. London: Granada Publishing Ltd., 1982.

———. *Sacred Waters*. London: Granada Publishing Ltd., 1985.

Dillon, Myles. *Early Irish Literature*. Chicago: University of Chicago Press, 1948.

Ferris, Helen. *Favorite Poems Old and New*. Garden City, N.Y.: Doubleday and Company, Inc., 1957.

Gimbutas, Marija. *The Goddesses and Gods of Old Europe 7000-3500 B.C.* Los Angeles: University of California Press, 1974.

Harley, J. L., and D. H. Lewis, eds. "The Flora and Vegetation of Britain," in *New Phytologist Trust*. New York: Academic Press, 1985.

Herm, Gerhard. *The Celts*. New York: St. Martin's Press, 1976.

Jacobi, Jolanda, ed. *Paracelsus, Selected Writings*, Bollingen Series XXVIII. New York: Pantheon Books, 1958.

Judge, William Q. *The Bhagavad-Gita*. Los Angeles: The Theosophy Company, 1971.

Kinsella, Thomas, trans. *Tain Bo Cuailnge*. London: Oxford University Press, 1970.

MacNeill, Eoin. "On the Calendar of Coligny." *Eriu*, Vol X, 1926–28: 1-67.

Markale, Jean. *Women of the Celts*. Rochester, Vt.: Inner Traditions International, 1986.

Matthews, Caitlin. *The Elements of the Celtic Tradition*. Longmead, Shaftsbury, U.K.: Element Books Ltd., 1989.

————, and John Matthews. *The Western Way*. New York: Arkana, Routledge and Kegan Paul Inc., 1986.

Merry, Eleanor C. *The Flaming Door*. Edinburgh: Floris Books, 1983.

Murphy, Gerard, ed. *Early Irish Lyrics: Eighth to Twelfth Century*. London: Oxford University Press, 1962.

Murray, Liz, and Colin Murray. *The Celtic Tree Oracle*. New York: St. Martin's Press, 1988.

Piggott, Stuart. *The Druids*. New York: Thames and Hudson, 1986.

Rees, Alwyn, and Brinley Rees. *Celtic Heritage*. New York: Thames and Hudson, 1989.

Ross, Anne. *Pagan Celtic Britain*. New York: Columbia University Press, 1967.

————, and Michael Cyprien. *A Traveller's Guide to Celtic Britain*. Boston: Historical Times Incorporated, 1985.

Sharp, E. A., and J. Matthay, eds. *Lyra Celtica*. Edinburgh: John Grant, 1932.

Squire, Charles. *Celtic Myth and Legend: Poetry and Romance*. Van Nuys, Calif.: Newcastle Publishing Co. Inc., 1975.

Stone, Merlin. *Ancient Mirrors of Womanhood*. Boston: Unitarian Universalist Association of Congregations, 1984.

Untermeyer, Louis. *A Treasury of Great Poems*. New York: Simon and Schuster, 1942.

Williams, Oscar, ed. *Immortal Poems of the English Language*. New York: Washington Square Press, 1965.

MAGICAL

Beyerl, Paul. *The Master Book of Herbalism*. Custer, Wash.: Phoenix Publishing Inc., 1984.

Cunningham, Scott. *Cunningham's Encyclopedia of Magical Herbs*. St. Paul, Minn.: Llewellyn Publications, 1986.

————. *Magical Herbalism: The Secret Craft of the Wise*. St. Paul, Minn.: Llewellyn Publications, 1986.

Hopman, Ellen Evert. *Tree Medicine, Tree Magic*. Custer, Wash.: Phoenix Publishing Inc., 1991.

Hurley, Phillip. *Herbal Alchemy*. Chicago: Lotus Publications, 1977.

Kerr, Ralph Whiteside. *Herbalism Through the Ages*. Supreme Grand Lodge of Amroc, San Jose, Calif.: 1969.

Riva, Anna. *The Modern Herbal Spellbook*. Los Angeles: International Imports, 1988.

Ryall, Rhiannon. *West Country Magic*. Custer, Wash.: Phoenix Publishing Inc., 1989.

HERBAL

BOOKS

Barefoot Doctor's Manual. Seattle, Wash.: Madrona Publishers, 1977.

Culbreth, David. *A Manual of Materia Medica and Pharmacology*. Philadelphia: Lea and Febiger, 1927.

Culpeper, Nicholas. *Culpeper's Color Herbal*. Edited by David Potterton. New York: Sterling Publishing Co., 1983.

Grieve, M. *A Modern Herbal*. New York: Dover Publishing Inc., 1982.

Harley, J. L., and D. H. Lewis, eds. "The Flora and Vegetation of Britain," in *New Phytologist Trust*. New York: Academic Press, 1985.

Hurley, Phillip. *Herbal Alchemy*. Chicago: Lotus Publications, 1977.

Junius, Manfred M. *Practical Handbook of Plant Alchemy*. Rochester, Vt.: Healing Arts Press, 1985.

Leroi, Rita. *An Anthroposophical Approach to Cancer*. Anthroposophical Therapy and Hygiene Association, 1973.

Lust, John. *The Herb Book*. New York: Bantam Books, 1983.

Meyer, Joseph E. *The Herbalist*. Edited by Clarence Meyer. 1975.

Millspaugh, Charles F. *American Medicinal Plants*. New York: Dover Publishing Inc., 1974.

Shook, Edward E. *Advanced Treatise on Herbology*. Beaumont, Calif.: Trinity Center Press, 1978.

Tierra, Michael. *Planetary Herbology*. Santa Fe: Lotus Press, 1988.

Treben, Maria. *Health Through God's Pharmacy*. Austria: Wilhelm Ennsthaler, Steyr, 1983.

Weed, Susun S. *Wisewoman Herbal for the Childbearing Year*. Woodstock N.Y.: Ash Tree Publishing, 1985.

Wyman, Donald. *Wyman's Gardening Encyclopedia*. New York: Macmillan Publishing Co., 1978.

JOURNAL ARTICLES

Aufmkolk, M., J. C. Ingbar, K. Kubota, S. M. Amir, S. H. Ingbar. "Extracts and Auto-Oxidized Constituents of Certain Plants Inhibit the Receptor-

Binding and the Biological Activity of Graves' Immunoglobulins," *Endocrinology* 116: (1985): 1687–93.

Embroden, W. "The Sacred Journey in Dynastic Egypt: Shamanistic Trance in the Context of the Narcotic Water Lily and the Mandrake," *Journal of Psychoactive Drugs* I: (1989): 61–75.

Hartwell, J. L. "Plants Used Against Cancer: A Survey," *Lloydia* 34: (1971): 204–55.

Honda, G., Tosirisuk, V., Tabata, M. "Isolation of an Antidermatophytic, Tryptanthrin, from Indigo Plants, Polygonum tinctorium and Isatis tinctoria," *Planta Medica* 38: (1980): 275–6.

Oncology: International Journal of Cancer Research and Treatment (special issue on mistletoe), December 1986.

Kessel, A. "'Mandrax'—No Significant Side Effects," *Medical Journal of Australia* 2: (1971): 166.

Lee, H., and Lin, J. Y. "Anti-Mutagenic Activity of Extracts from Anti-Cancer Drugs in Chinese Medicine," *Mutation Research* 204: (1988): 229–34.

Nuland, S. B. "The Origins of Anesthesia," *Connecticut Medicine* 48: (1984): 171–4.

O'Rourke, M. G. "'Mandrax'—No Significant Side Effects," *Medical Journal of Australia* 2: (1971): 873.

Ross, C. H. "Granny's Herbs and the Third Crusade," *Anesthesia and Analgesia* 50: (1971): 609–11.

Swiatek, L. "Phenolic Acids of Underground Parts of Scrophularia Nodosa L.," *Polish Journal of Pharmacology and Pharmacy* 25: (1973): 461–4.

Tabba, H. D., R. S. Chang, and K. M. Smith. "Isolation, Purification and Partial Characterization of Prunellin, an Anti-HIV Component from Aqueous Extracts of Prunella Vulgaris," *Antiviral Research* II: (1989): 263–73.

Weston, F. "'Mandrax'—No Significant Side Effects," *Medical Journal of Australia* 2: (1971): 446.

HOMEOPATHIC

Boericke, William. *Materia Medica with Repertory*. Philadephia, Pa.: Boericke and Tafel, 1927.

Cummings, Stephen, and Dana Ullman. *Everybody's Guide to Homeopathic Medicines*. Los Angeles: Jeremy P. Tarcher, Inc., 1984.

Danciger, Elizabeth. *Homeopathy: From Alchemy to Medicine*. Rochester, Vt.: Healing Arts Press, 1988.

Koehler, Gerhard. *Handbook of Homeopathy*. Rochester, Vt.: Healing Arts Press, 1989.

Smith, Trevor. *Homeopathic Medicine: A Doctor's Guide to Remedies for Common Ailments*. Rochester, Vt.: Healing Arts Press, 1989.

Plant Index

Lady's slipper, 87, 175

Larkspur. *See* Delphinium

Lavender (*Lavandula vera*), 45, 63, 71, 94, 124, 131, 145, 171, 190

Lemon verbena (*Lippia citriodora*), 171–72

Licorice (*Glycyrrhiza glabra*), 146, 172

Linseed. *See* Flax

Lotus (*Nelumbo nucifera*), 154–55, 172

Madder (*Rubia tinctorum*), 90, 94, 131

Maidenhair fern (*Adiantum capillus-veneris*), 84–85, 124

Male fern (*Dryopteris filix-mas*), 71, 94, 133

Mandrake (*Mandragora officinalis*), 95–98, 125, 133, 143, 155, 181

Maple (*Acer* spp.), 172–73, 191

Marigold (*Calendula officinalis*), 60, 81, 85–86, 121

Marjoram (*Origanum majorana*), 155, 173

Marshmallow (*Althea* sp.), 86, 121, 126, 127, 131

Meadowsweet (*Spiraea ulmaris*), 61, 72, 98–99, 131, 173

Melilot (*Melilotus officinalis*), 181

Milk thistle (*Sylybum marianum*), 89

Milkweed (*Asclepias syriaca*), 86, 191

Mint (*Mentha sativa*), 99–100, 126, 127

Mistletoe (*Viscum album*), 12, 31, 36, 72, 79, 100–104, 105, 106, 121, 131, 143, 173

Monkshood. *See* Aconite

Moonwort (*Botrychium lunaria*), 85

Mosses, 106–7

Mugwort (*Artemisia vulgaris*), 71, 72, 94, 126

Mulberry, 37, 97, 125, 131, 191–92

Mullein (*Verbascum thapsus*), 26–27, 44, 133

Myrrh (*Commiphora myrrha*), 44, 86–87, 131, 155

Nightshade (*Solanum dulcamara*), 27

Oak (*Quercus* spp.), 23–24, 59, 65, 80, 101, 104–6, 130, 131, 135, 143–44, 166. *See also* Acorns

Oats (*Avena sativa*), 80, 125, 131

Olibanum. *See* Frankincense

Orchid root (*Orchis* spp.), 61, 127, 173

Parsley (*Carum petroselinum*), 156, 192

Pasque flower (*Anemone pulsatilla*), 156–57

Passion flower (*Passiflora incanata*), 87, 121, 175

Pennyroyal (*Mentha pulegium*), 25, 72, 126, 127, 157–58

Peppermint, 69, 78, 84, 175

Periwinkle (*Vinca minor*), 158

Pine (*Pinus* spp.), 37, 73, 101, 133, 144, 158–59, 181–82

Plantain (*Plantago lanceolta*), 94, 126, 127, 133, 182

Poison oak, 110, 182

Poke root (*Phylotacca americana*), 67

Poplar (*Populus balsamifera*), 101, 131, 133, 159

Poppy (*Papaver somniferum*), 97, 122, 123, 133

Primrose. *See* Cowslip

Pulsatilla. *See* Pasque flower

Pumpkin (*Cucurbita pepo*), 27–28, 123

Queen-of-the-Meadow. *See* Meadowsweet

Quince (*Cydonia vulgaris*), 37, 133, 173–74

Rose (*Rosa* spp.), 45, 51–52, 61, 63, 73, 87, 122, 123, 126, 127, 131, 145, 174

Rosemary (*Rosmarinus officinalis*), 144, 159, 174, 182–83

Rowan (*Sorbus aucuparia*), 54, 62, 76, 105, 135, 144, 183

Subject Index

Abscesses, 60, 78, 153
Aengus Og, 39, 47
Alchemy, herbal, 119–20
Alcoholism, 24, 40, 50, 154, 170, 175
All Hallows Eve. *See* Samhain
Anemia, 78, 92, 153, 192, 193
Antibiotics, 25, 34, 50, 71, 84, 108–9, 113, 152, 153, 161, 170, 180, 188
Antifungals, 25, 115–16, 178
Aphrodisiacs, 78, 110, 169–70
Arteriosclerosis, 59, 102
Arthritis, 37, 45, 58, 99, 159, 162, 163, 178, 181, 192
Asthma, 69, 73, 86, 87, 100, 103, 114, 141, 142, 156, 161, 162, 167, 170, 172, 178, 183, 188, 190, 192
Astringents, 23, 28, 48, 111–12
Athlete's foot, 25, 115–16

Bards, 6–8
Baths, 48, 49, 51, 60, 71, 72, 80, 94, 111, 114, 140, 141, 142, 144, 152, 155, 158, 170, 187
Beltaine, 53–56
Bile, 65
Bladder tonics, 25, 33, 35, 49, 62, 63, 68, 73, 79, 80, 110, 112, 145, 159, 163, 168, 182, 188

Bleeding, 23, 60, 102, 107, 112, 115, 154, 162, 175. *See also* Hemorrhages
Blood pressure, 59, 102, 108–9, 112, 127, 153, 168, 172, 182
Blood purifiers, 58, 60, 69, 89, 92, 93, 94, 179, 192
Boand, 47, 56
Boils, 78, 181, 188
Bone healing, 88, 94, 191
Bonfires, 21, 30, 39, 55–56, 65, 66, 71, 93–94
Breast cancer, 93, 102
Breast milk, 28, 34, 35, 38, 69, 73, 89, 161, 168. *See also* Childbirth; Pregnancy
Brighid, 31–32, 38–39
Bronchitis, 27, 35, 37, 69, 78, 84, 86, 141, 142, 145, 155, 156, 160, 167, 178–81, 188, 189
Bruises, 93, 113, 114, 142, 157, 169, 178
Burns, 41, 42, 43, 73, 85, 92, 93, 157, 159, 187

Cailleach, 83
Cancer, 45, 49, 50, 57, 58, 60, 62–63, 70, 73, 89, 93, 101–2, 156, 160, 163. *See also* Tumors
Candlemas. *See* Imbolc/Oimealg
Cataracts, 70, 81

For Further Reading

PEOPLE OF THE EARTH

The New Pagans Speak Out
Interviews with Margot Adler, Starhawk,
Susun Weed, Z. Budapest, and Many Others
ELLEN EVERT HOPMAN AND LAWRENCE BOND • ISBN 0-89281-559-0 • $19.95 PB

The authors examine the origins and activities of modern Paganism, and provide a forum for a variety of Pagan leaders to share their beliefs and practices. From Margot Adler, NPR reporter and author of *Drawing Down the Moon* to Oberon Zell, founder of the Church of All Worlds, the people interviewed here express the rich diversity of modern Paganism and provide a personal view of one of today's most dynamic spiritual movements.

THE CELTIC BOOK OF DAYS

A Guide to Celtic Spirituality and Wisdom
CAITLÍN MATTHEWS
ISBN 0-89281-565-5 • COLOR ILLUSTRATIONS THROUGHOUT • $24.95 HARDCOVER

With the delicate beauty of an illuminated manuscript, this richly illustrated volume features thoughtful selections from Celtic myth, poetry, prayers, and customs for each day of the year. Organized around the Celtic calendar, it is strongly linked to the seasonal turning of the year, and draws from both Christian and Pagan traditions. This elegant book is a treasury that you will turn to again and again for quiet thoughts of inspiration that bring the rich traditions of Celtic art and spirituality into daily life.

EARTH MAGIC

A Wisewoman's Guide to Herbal, Astrological, and Other Folk Wisdom
CLAIRE NAHMAD • ISBN 0-89281-424-1 • $12.95 PAPERBACK

"The author draws upon the rich symbolism of Celtic mythology to provide an introduction to a holistic feminine philosophy steeped in the Druidic past. Chapters are organized around the signs of the zodiac and convey a mixture of esoteric information and practical wisdom. An interesting look at an alternative spiritual path." **Library Journal**

GREEN PHARMACY

The History and Evolution of Western Herbal Medicine

BARBARA GRIGGS • ISBN 0-89281-427-6 • $19.95 PAPERBACK

Explore the history of medicine beginning with evidence of Neanderthal plant medicine and proceeding through centuries and civilizations, touching on the people and events that shaped the course of medicine up to the present time. The author shows that the popularity of herbal therapy in any given period is related to cyclical failures of organized medicine, when treatment becomes more severe than the disease.

"…a modern classic… insight into the trials and tribulations, the pitfalls and rewards, and the history and future of drug therapy from nature."

Norman R. Farnsworth, M.D.
Professor of Pharmacognosy
University of Illinois Medical Center

THE GREEN WITCH HERBAL

Restoring Nature's Magic in Home, Health, and Beauty Care

BARBARA GRIGGS • ISBN 0-89281-496-9 • $14.95 PAPERBACK

For centuries, the "green witch" was honored for her extensive knowledge of plant properties, and the herbs and flowers in her garden supplied medicines, perfumes, and cleansers. That knowledge can be yours with this modern sourcebook of herbal wisdom. Full of practical advice and fascinating historical insights, it provides information that will enable you to create your own personal, health, and home care products.

THE CELTS

Uncovering the Historic and Mythic Origins of Western Culture

JEAN MARKALE • ISBN 0-89281-413-6 • $14.95 PAPERBACK

"Markale has created a vivid picture—poetic and philosophical—of this deeply spiritual people. Here are the prophecies of Merlin and the druids, Celtic mythology, the Britons and Bretons, the Celtic Christian church, the history of the Gaels. This is a well-researched, erudite study of Celticism and its core beliefs."

The Book Reader

PLANTS OF THE GODS

Their Sacred, Healing, and Hallucinogenic Powers
RICHARD EVANS SCHULTES AND ALBERT HOFMANN
ISBN 0-89281-406-3 • $22.95 PAPERBACK • 400 COLOR AND BLACK AND WHITE ILLUSTRATIONS

Two eminent researchers detail the use of hallucinogenic plants in the shamanic healing rites of indigenous cultures throughout history and around the world. Dr. Schultes is retired from Harvard University where he was a Jeffrey Professor of Biology and Director of the Botanical Museum. Dr. Hofmann, the discoverer of LSD, is the retired director of the Pharmaceutical-Chemical Research Laboratory of Sandoz, Ltd. Switzerland.

"...an extraordinary blend of botany, ethnobotany, chemistry, history, mythology, and art. A visual, spiritual, and intellectual feast, this is the best book ever written on hallucinogenic plants." **Dr. Mark Plotkin**
Conservation International

WOMEN HEALERS

Portraits of Herbalists, Physicians, and Midwives
ELISABETH BROOKE • 0-89281-548-5 • $12.95 PAPERBACK

Drawing on primary sources for her revisionist history, the author highlights important contributions of women healers from ancient times to the present.

"Brooke's women healers are gentle and compassionate people, less concerned with the brilliance of developing technology than with the care of the patient."
The Daily Mail

THE PRACTICAL HANDBOOK OF PLANT ALCHEMY

An Herbalist's Guide to Preparing Medicinal Essences, Tinctures, and Elixirs
MANFRED JUNIUS • ISBN 0-89281-485-3 • $16.95 PAPERBACK

The author describes in detail nearly forgotten but highly valuable alchemical methods for preparing plant remedies. While ordinary tinctures and infusions use only a part of the great curative potential of plants, the methods of plant alchemy "open" the medicinal plants completely, bringing forth their more powerful healing properties.

THE PAGAN BOOK OF DAYS

A Guide to the Festivals, Traditions, and Sacred Days of the Year
NIGEL PENNICK
ISBN 0-89281-369-5 • BLACK AND WHITE ILLUSTRATIONS THROUGHOUT • $9.95 PAPERBACK

This fascinating almanac contains an entry for each day of the year, drawn from rituals and celebrations of the ancient Greek, Roman, Celtic, Anglo-Saxon, Wiccan, and Norse traditions. The author is an authority on ancient belief systems, and he provides details on the Eight Stations of the Year, holy days of the ancient gods and goddesses, auspicious and inauspicious days, the movements of the planets, and lunar and solar calendars from now through the millenium.

WOMEN IN CELTIC MYTH

Tales of Extraordinary Women from Ancient Celtic Traditions
MOYRA CALDECOTT • ISBN 0-89281-357-1 • $12.95 PAPERBACK

These intriguing stories—some more than 3,000 years old—focus on the women of Celtic mythology, from formidable women warriors to the gentle women who guided others to spiritual wisdom.

CELEBRATING THE GREAT MOTHER

A Handbook of Earth-Honoring Activities for Parents and Children
CAIT JOHNSON AND MAURA D. SHAW • ISBN 0-89281-550-7 • $16.95 ILLUSTRATED PAPERBACK

The activities collected in this delightful book will bring children into the rituals celebrating seasonal cycles and help reclaim the spiritual roots of our holidays. Create a family altar; make dream pillows; cast bean runes; gather smudge sticks; play games; keep journals. Here you will find a wealth of enjoyable, earth-honoring activities to inspire children of all ages.

These and other Inner Traditions titles are available at many fine bookstores or, to order from the publisher, send a check or money order for the total amount, payable to Inner Traditions, plus $3.50 shipping for the first book and $1.00 for each additional book to:

Inner Traditions, P.O. Box 388, Rochester, VT 05767